Jo[...]

Donald Andrew
Born June 25, 1968

24 00

9988

AWAKE AND AWARE

AWAKE AND AWARE

PARTICIPATING IN CHILDBIRTH
THROUGH PSYCHOPROPHYLAXIS

IRWIN CHABON, M.D.

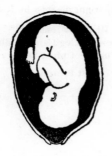

Introduction by Heinz L. Luschinsky, M.D.
President, the American Society for
Psychoprophylaxis in Obstetrics

DELACORTE PRESS / NEW YORK

The drawings in Chapter II are renderings of life-size sculptures prepared by Dr. Robert L. Dickinson and Abram Belskie from thousands of hospital X-rays. Photographic reproductions of the twenty-four sculptures are published as *The Birth Atlas* by the Maternity Center Association.

FOR ADY

CONTENTS

CONTENTS

Preface

Even modest works such as this do not "just grow." They arise in response to a need, a need which someone recognizes. The need for *Awake and Aware* was recognized by Dr. Benjamin Segal during his tenure as president of the American Society for Psychoprophylaxis in Obstetrics. He convinced the Dell Publishing Company that there was a need for a book, and it was then duly commissioned. Without Dr. Segal's vision and persistence there would be no ASPO and certainly no *Awake and Aware*. He willingly and cheerfully gave of his time to review the manuscript during its preparation, and it has benefited greatly from his penetrating criticism. ASPO as an organization has grown to its present stature as a result of his leadership. All of us now involved in the practice of psychoprophylaxis and its dissemination are indebted to Dr. Segal.

It would be impossible for me to pinpoint the source of every idea expressed in this book. However, there are several people to whom I am particularly indebted. I

9

received my specialty training in obstetrics and gynecology under Dr. Martin L. Stone, Professor and Chair-
man, Department of Obstetrics and Gynecology, New
York Medical College–Metropolitan Medical Center. It
was with his assistance that the Prenatal Education Program, which includes training in psychoprophylaxis, was
begun in September of 1960 at that institution.

I am especially grateful to Dr. Alfred Tanz, who encouraged my interest in this approach to childbirth during my residency training and taught me much. When
he was organizing the Prenatal Education Program in
1960 he invited me to associate with him in the conduct
of the program, and we have worked together in the
training of mothers ever since.

My association with Mrs. Elizabeth Bing, head of
teacher training for ASPO, began at the Prenatal Education Program in 1960 and has been very rewarding for
me. Most of what I know of the practical implementation of psychoprophylactic techniques I learned from
this most effective and charming lady.

The religious points of view presented in this book
were reviewed by clergy of the different faiths. Dr.
George Landes and Dr. Paul Lehmann of Union Theological Seminary kindly gave me their help. The
Roman Catholic view was explained to me and checked,
once inserted in the text, by my good friend Father J.
Joseph Hoffman, S.J. My fellow naval reservist Rabbi
Nisson Shulman, of Congregation Sons of Israel, Yon-
kers, N. Y., reviewed the presentation of the Jewish point
of view.

I am very grateful to Mr. Robert Yellin for his mar-
velous photography. Through his mastery of his me-

dium he has expressed more than I could ever hope to convey with words.

Words, of course, mean manuscript, and manuscript means editor. To Miss Joanne Dolinar fell the unhappy task of taking my raw material and converting it into something readable. She has succeeded despite the raw. ness of some of the material. I greatly appreciate her patience and skill in editing the manuscript.

Everyone has someone in his life who occupies for him a rather special position—not a parent, not just a friend, not just a colleague: someone who is none of these quite and yet all of them at once; someone whose influence cannot be measured, but is nonetheless there. For me this special someone has been Dr. Abner I. Weisman. His encouragement, sharp and incisive criticism, honesty and sincere friendship have enriched me and to a great extent made this book a reality.

Finally, no series of acknowledgments could be complete without a special thanks to those many mothers who have permitted me the profound pleasure of assisting them in the birth of their children. It is really their happiness that has inspired this book.

I. C.

AWAKE AND AWARE

Introduction

To be awake, aware, and to participate in childbirth has become the battle cry of a determined group of young parents—much to the discomfort of the majority of obstetricians, nurses, and hospital administrators who cherish the good old "routine."

The reasons for our present-day routine date back to the turn of the century when hospital delivery replaced home delivery. This step was then dictated by a very great infant and maternal mortality from hemorrhage and infection during home delivery. Physical prenatal care, as we know it today, was instituted around this time. The transfer of childbirth from home to hospital corresponded to a medical need but was bought at a price. The healthy pregnant woman became a patient, a creature carrying a uterus out of which a fetus had to be removed under sterile precautions. Much greater safety for mother and child was achieved at the price of complete spatial and emotional isolation of the mother from her husband, her familiar surroundings, and her child.

Yes, even the child was stabled away from the mother in a nursery for bacteriological reasons and encouraged to drink cow's milk.

Should we not ask sixty years later whether these reasons for isolation of the woman during labor and after delivery are still valid in the age of the sulfa drug, the antibiotic, the blood bank and the safe Caesarian section? Should we not ask whether it is sufficient to supervise merely the physical aspects of a pregnancy and to neglect the pregnant woman and her emotional needs? Should we not ask whether it is right to delegate childbirth to the obstetrician?

In nonindustrialized cultures, a pregnant woman is surrounded by persons of all ages who regard her problems as their problems. In our Western civilization, however, a young woman and man, both away from their parental homes, are likely to face their problems alone, in need of guidance, but not finding it. Physical supervision alone is not enough. Clinic patients rebel against the rigid physical orientation of our prenatal care in the large urban clinics by a stay-away strike. Hundreds of letters and innumerable telephone calls to the American Society for Psychoprophylaxis in Obstetrics (ASPO) are testimony that young mothers are no longer content with physical supervision alone. They want to prepare themselves actively for childbirth and not delegate all responsibility to the doctors.

Psychoprophylaxis is intellectual, physical, and emotional preparation for childbirth and parenthood. No longer is the young woman left to herself with her fears and anxieties as to what it will be like. She and her husband will be prepared for childbirth and she will be trained to cope with its stress by specific techniques. She will not be left alone in labor. Her husband will be with her and together they will witness the birth of their child.

Psychoprophylaxis not only respects the social bond between husband and wife but also the biological bond between mother and child. The mother should have her baby with her or have access to her baby at any time. This means rooming-in or open nursery. The hospital stay should be a learning situation for both parents so that they do not carry home what seems to be a strange bundle.

Among the thousands of hospitals in this country, we have but one at this moment which carries through all the principles of psychoprophylaxis—namely, St. Mary's Hospital in Evansville, Indiana, under the leadership of Sister Stella Mary.

Childbirth is beginning to wear a new face in America. Much of the pioneering work was done by enthusiastic women like Marjorie Karmel, author of the popular book *Thank You, Dr. Lamaze,* who experienced the method. In this tradition, volunteers of ASPO now answer letters, write brochures, arrange meetings, show films, talk to their friends, and, more important, they demand what they want from their obstetricians.

Dr. Chabon's book fills a real need because it describes psychoprophylaxis adapted to American conditions. This book is not meant only for the expectant mother. Dr. Chabon expressed to me what I believe to be fundamentally true: psychoprophylaxis starts at the cradle. We must reach the prospective mother before she is pregnant. This book should be on the reading list of every high-school or college course concerned with sex education, courtship, marriage and the family. Dr. Chabon himself has pioneered along these lines by giving lectures to teen-agers about pregnancy and showing them a movie depicting an actual birth. There was not a sneer or a snicker. There were open ears and open eyes and open hearts. Our young people are ready for the facts. Are we ready to give them?

The true meaning of psychoprophylaxis cannot be expressed better than by the mothers. In this book they speak of the deep and all-encompassing sense of fulfillment. "Giving birth was a feeling that I will never forget, and yet never be able to explain. It is a glow and yet it is more. Without the help of my husband and doctor, I often wonder whether I would have been equally successful."

"The child was incredible to behold, beautiful in every way, folded like a new butterfly." These mothers have understood that there is no greater joy than to give birth in dignity and surrounded by their loved ones.

These comments may sound too rhapsodic. Was there no pain? The Russian originators and the French School equate psychoprophylaxis to childbirth "without pain." One of our mothers had this to say: "Sure I had pain, but at no time did I suffer!"

Psychoprophylaxis is not for heroes or martyrs, is not a dogma or a key to heaven, is not a proving ground to assert one's femininity. It is simply a fine way to become a parent—the best I know.

HEINZ L. LUSCHINSKY, M.D.
President, the American Society for
Psychoprophylaxis in Obstetrics

Prologue

At 3:00 A.M. Mrs. Brown woke from a troubled sleep with a start. What was this ache she had in her back? What was this tightness that seized her abdomen? She knew, of course, that her baby was due, that she was supposed to "go into labor." But all she knew of labor was what she had heard. She was supposed to have labor pains, which would get worse and worse until the child was born. That undoubtedly was what this was!

As these thoughts raced through her mind, she became frightened. She had a vaginal discharge, which was tinged with blood. What was this? Was something wrong? Her doctor had given her instructions to call him when the labor pains were occurring every five minutes for one hour. She timed them and found that they were occurring every seven minutes. The doctor had said not to call—but these were severe pains. What to do? She called the doctor, who said that if she couldn't stand it at home to go on to the hospital, and he would be along.

She awakened her husband and told him what had happened. He too became upset and frightened. Was this really labor? Was she going to have the child to-night—this minute, perhaps? They dressed quickly and rushed to the hospital. The labor pains were now every three minutes, and of strong intensity. With each con-traction, Mrs. Brown moaned, writhed, clenched her fists and gritted her teeth. Was this how one had a baby?

At the hospital she was admitted, then crisply and efficiently taken in tow. Tearfully she bade her husband goodbye. Alone and frightened in the labor room, she begged for an injection. The doctor's magic needle soon put her out, and there was nothing left for her to do.

She awoke half a day later to find her abdomen flat and her bottom sore. It was all over. She was a mother. But what had happened? Where were those hours since the injection? Were they never to be hers? A child was brought to her. On its wrist and ankle were bands with a name and number. I guess this must be mine, she thought. Was it a boy or a girl? She felt she should have known. After all, it was *her* child.

At 3:00 A.M. Mrs. Green woke from a deep sleep. She slowly sat up in bed and gathered her wits about her. Her baby was due, and she had eagerly been anticipating the onset of labor. What was going on now? She felt a dull, slightly uncomfortable sensation in her lower back, and a periodic tightness of the abdomen occurring every seven or eight minutes. These must be contractions of early labor, she thought. She also had a profuse vaginal discharge, which seemed bloody. This must be the "bloody show." It seems just about what they taught us to expect in Prenatal Class, she thought. Well, that's good. This must be labor. It's not uncomfortable, so there's nothing to do just yet. The instructor had said not to begin using the breathing exercises for relief of discomfort until it became necessary.

Within an hour or so, contractions became well established, and she was able to time them easily. When they had been occurring every five minutes for some time, she called her doctor. He asked her how she was getting on—was she comfortable, did she need the breathing techniques yet? When it was apparent that all was going well, he told her to remain at home a bit longer and to call him in an hour.

She felt fine. She was in touch with her doctor, she understood her labor, and she had been trained to work with it and to help herself. Her husband understood too, and they both, with the help and guidance of their obstetrician, were managing just fine. She remained in touch with her doctor by phone, and she dealt with her contractions as she had been taught in the Prenatal Class in psychoprophylaxis.

Soon she was instructed to go to the hospital. Having visited the hospital before and seen the facilities and personnel, she knew where to go, what to do, whom to see. She was admitted, shaved, and given an enema. Then her husband was at her side. Together they worked with her labor, she performing the breathing exercises with each contraction, he coaching, calling the time, criticizing her performance, keeping her attention focused on her tasks.

Labor progressed normally and well, and soon the baby was ready to be born. The delivery team—mother-to-be, husband, and doctor—now moved to the delivery room. Mrs. Green was awake and completely aware of what was going on. More important, her active participation in and cooperation with the process of her child-birth made her the star player in this greatest of human dramas. She worked, the doctor advised, her husband encouraged and supported. From this a baby was born, and all were present and could witness its emergence into the world. Seconds after birth, this child first felt the warmth of its mother's love as she held it to her. Seconds after birth, this child basked in the radiance of its father's face and heart. From the moment of birth, the family—father, mother, child—came into being as a unit, and so they would exist henceforth.

This mother did not need to be told the sex of her child. She brought it forth and saw for herself. She did not need to examine a number on a bracelet to know that this was her child. She watched the bracelet being put on. This mother and child did not need to be introduced to each other by the nursery attendant. They met each other at the instant of birth.

I

What Is Psychoprophylaxis?

In the United States today, childbirth can be conducted in a variety of ways—as with much else in the "affluent society." The two births described in the prologue represent the extremes: an unprepared woman relieved with an amnesiac and delivered by her obstetrician, and a thoroughly prepared woman delivering her child with the skill and guidance of her doctor and the help of her husband. The first method, commonly known as being "put out," is probably the most frequently employed in metropolitan areas of this country. But, as the American woman becomes more sophisticated, she seeks to recover childbirth as her own possession. For some fifty years it has belonged to the doctors. Today's young women, in ever-increasing numbers, look upon childbirth as one of the most precious of life's experiences. They want to be awake and aware; they want to participate actively in the birth of their children. And they want to share this experience with their husbands.

Such active participation in childbirth requires extensive and thorough preparation—preparation in a method that is realistic, not fanciful; and practical, not merely theoretical. Such a method is psychoprophylaxis. Its theoretical basis is sound, its implementation is simple, and it works.

Psychoprophylaxis is usually categorized with other techniques that have similar objectives as "natural childbirth." This term is alarmingly inaccurate. What exactly is natural childbirth? The meaning of the word "childbirth" is obvious. And "natural" is also an easy word— or is it?

In lower animals, birth patterns are instinctive, and therefore are "natural." Lower animals act and react as they were *constructed* to act and react. They have no ability to control or alter their behavior. They mate instinctively—their urge usually governed by hormones —and become pregnant. As the lower mammals approach term and its associated labor, nesting instincts are aroused, and the pregnant animal selects a location for her delivery and gathers soft materials to make a comfortable nest in which to deliver her young. When labor comes along, the pregnant mammal repairs to her nest, delivers her young, bites the cord, cleans the young, puts them to her breast, and eats the placentas. This is truly *natural* childbirth. The entire behavior pattern is unlearned and is repeated time after time in the same species in a predictable fashion.

The biological aspects of human childbirth are also "natural"—coitus, resultant fertilization, development and growth of the new human being within the reproductive organs of the mother, and finally the termination of the pregnancy through the mechanism of labor, the uterine contractions that press the child through the birth canal. But the one uniquely human quality—abstract thought and the associated ability to communicate—makes natural childbirth, in the true meaning of the term, impossible for human beings. There lives not the woman who can respond to pregnancy, labor and delivery on the instinctive level, who can give birth in a given, predetermined fashion over which she has no control and which she would repeat action for action in subsequent pregnancies.

The great anthropologist Margaret Mead has studied childbirth customs thoroughly. She has concluded that even in preliterate human societies, attitudes toward and behavior in childbirth are *socially* determined. Take an Eskimo baby, transpose her to a tribe of African head-hunters, and raise her there. She will have her babies like a headhunter woman rather than an Eskimo woman, for it was among the headhunters that she *learned* how. A cat, however, will have its young in the same predictable cat fashion whether raised by Eskimos, headhunters, Americans or Europeans.

Within limits, each woman will experience childbirth in a roughly predictable fashion, depending upon the social grouping from which she comes and in which she has *learned* how one behaves under given circumstances. The corollary is that human behavior patterns in childbirth can be *unlearned* as well, and new patterns—more or less efficient than the old—can be substituted.

Returning to the original question, what then is natural childbirth? As we have seen, the term is an unfortunate one. It was coined by a doctor, Grantley Dick-Read, who believed that childbirth without analgesic medications and anesthesia and with minimal medical interference was most desirable for the infant under normal circumstances—a contention with which no one disagrees. He felt that the mother's participation in and awareness of the entire labor and delivery are most important—that childbirth is one of the most profound emotional experiences of a woman's life, and that conscious participation in the process will create a mother-child relationship that is healthier from the beginning. Dick-Read devised a series of exercises to train women how to help cope with their labors and how to deliver their children while fully conscious. In fact, the first book he wrote on the subject was titled *Natural Childbirth*. The term caught on and has come to mean any method of preparation and training for labor that eliminates or reduces the need for pain-relieving medications.

Many philosophies and new methods have been introduced since Dick-Read began writing in 1932. One of these is psychoprophylaxis. This method was introduced in the Soviet Union and was brought to the West by Dr. Fernand Lamaze of Paris in 1952. Shortly thereafter it was popularized in the United States by the late Marjorie Karmel in her book *Thank You, Dr. Lamaze*.

Psychoprophylaxis proved superior to previous methods. A mother trained in the psychoprophylactic method is taught to understand the physiological and psychological processes involved in pregnancy, labor and delivery. She is taught to view childbirth as something for which nature has ingeniously prepared her and which, therefore, should not be unbearable. At the same time she learns a series of exercises and breathing techniques to help her work with her uterine contractions and to participate actively and effectively in the expulsion phase of labor—the actual delivery. Education and training are available to American women in classes that have sprung up throughout the country (see listing, p. 167), and many women have successfully used the method on their own, without benefit of formal classroom instruction.

What is most attractive about psychoprophylaxis to many women is that it permits the husband to play an active supportive role in the childbirth complex. In the United States he can choose to attend classes with her and serve as her coach for the exercise and breathing techniques. Because he is trained in what his wife is to do, he is permitted to remain in the labor room with her to encourage and direct her work. In an ever increasing number of hospitals he continues his support in the delivery room during the actual birth.

How does psychoprophylaxis work? Childbirth, no matter how normal, is associated with some degree of discomfort. How much discomfort is appropriate, and, more importantly, how much is tolerable? This is the great variable. In any given woman, the degree of discomfort caused by uterine contractions—labor pains—is influenced by two important factors: first, the actual physiologically transmitted discomfort (the strength of the signal sent from the uterus to the brain, which may be interpreted as pain); and second, the behavioral response to this signal once it has been interpreted by the brain. Influences can be exerted both to minimize the strength of the signal received in the brain and to alter the behavioral response to whatever signal is received.

The exercises taught by the psychoprophylactic method are based on what is known as the theory of conditioned reflexes. The method takes advantage of the fact that the brain can accept, integrate, interpret and emanate only *one* set of signals at a time. If the strongest set of signals arriving at the brain comes from the uterus and is interpreted as a labor pain, the forthcoming behavioral response, in keeping with such an unpleasant interpretation, is apt to be writhing, moaning, groaning, and perhaps weeping. But if at the instant of the uterine contraction a series of actions is initiated that requires for its successful execution stronger signals than those the uterus sends, then the uterine signals of necessity assume second place and the conscious perception of the uterine contraction diminishes markedly. The exercises of psychoprophylaxis provide the strong set of stimuli necessary to take precedence over the signals from the uterine contractions.

A more thorough discussion of this theory will appear in later pages. But it must be stressed that psychoprophylaxis is not merely a method of dealing with uterine contractions; it is a method of total preparation for childbirth. Total preparation means learning what the process of having a baby involves, removing superstition and misinformation, and absorbing valid, scientific information. Knowing what is happening to her helps a woman accept the phenomena without undue excitement or fear. Such knowledge also permits a woman to work effectively with her labor. For example, most pregnant women, whether sedated or not, are instructed to "bear down" and push out their babies in the final moments of labor. The reflex response of the untrained mother is eventually effective. The coordinated, consciously controlled expulsive effort of the trained mother, however, is more effective and leads to easier and more rapid expulsion of the child. The trained mother knows her body, knows which muscles to contract and which to relax. She knows *how* to have a baby. The untrained mother, on the other hand, is permitted to proceed on the mythical assumption that women are born knowing how to have babies. Nothing, of course, could be further from the truth.

Why deliver one's own child if the obstetrician can take care of everything? Why work hard for six weeks preparing for childbirth when one injection can remove the conscious mother from the scene?

That there is a practical medical value in prepared childbirth is unquestionable. No one would deny that the safest method of childbirth for both mother and baby is normally one without drugs or surgical interference. A normal birth, by definition, will be effected without harming mother or child if nothing is done to or for the mother. Most interference in the normal birth process is done to *enhance maternal comfort*. Normal healthy childbirth will proceed to its normal healthy conclusion even if the mother is uncomfortable.

The most commonly used method of enhancing maternal comfort is administering drugs: analgesics, which relieve pain, and anesthetics, which deaden all sensation. The most common analgesic drug used during labor is meperidine (Demerol). Administered properly, there is little risk, but should the baby be born too soon after a fairly heavy analgesic dose to the mother, the possibility exists of a "sleepy" baby, affected by the drug like the mother. This child may be slow to begin breathing and thus may not function ideally in those important minutes after birth, the first few minutes on its own.

All anesthetic techniques for delivery, if they are truly anesthetic, impair the mother's ability to work with her contractions to help expel the child. With general anesthesia (gas) the mother is unconscious and thus cannot cooperate at all. Conduction techniques (spinal, saddle, caudal), although permitting maternal consciousness, cause a certain amount of temporary muscle paralysis, again preventing maternal participation. The obstetrician must then supplant the mother—the child must be delivered with obstetrical forceps.

The administration of drugs, although a thoroughly tried technique, is never completely without hazard to the mother and child. It is true that the chances of an untoward occurrence are small, and it is argued that drugs can be used freely in the normal birth precisely because the incidence of difficulties is so slight. However, it is known that in normal instances birth will be effected without detriment to mother or child if no drugs are given to the mother. Is, then, the rare complication from analgesia or anesthesia acceptable? There is no question that when obstetrical disease is present, measures must be taken even though there may be intrinsic risks. The risks must be balanced: If the treatment is less risky than the disease, it is employed; if it is not, it is discarded. But most interference in the birth process is for the sake of maternal comfort, not medical necessity.

One of the chief advantages of psychoprophylaxis is that it provides a relatively comfortable way to have a baby—without the risks that drugs and surgical interference brings. It must be stressed that psychoprophylaxis does not promise complete elimination of all the discomfort of childbirth for all women. It does, however, reduce discomfort to quite manageable proportions for most trained women, and for many it can eliminate the discomfort totally.

The reason that psychoprophylaxis is becoming more

and more popular, however, is not only this unques-
tioned medical advantage. A growing number of women
want to know what childbirth is all about, to have their
very own memories of having delivered their children.
Psychoprophylaxis does not promise a spiritual uplifting
or an automatically improved mother-child relationship,
as does the Dick-Read method. It offers the mother a way
to experience the basic miracle of life, and she can then
place her own value judgment upon it. For many women,
it is a profound emotional experience; for others, it is
merely a convenient way to have a baby.

Psychoprophylaxis is neither a display of heroics nor a
contest against milligrams of injected analgesic. It is a
way to be awake, aware, and fully participating during
childbirth; a way to have, for one's very own, the childbirth experience. But it is not easy. The word "labor"
was applied to the childbirth process because it is hard
physical work. So is preparing for labor. One can decide
only after becoming a mother whether it was worth
while. Without preparation, there is no decision, no
evaluation, no experience. There is a pregnancy, a void,
and motherhood. With psychoprophylaxis that void can
be filled, if one chooses.

There has been a great to-do in both the lay and the
medical press over preparation for childbirth and the
use of psychoprophylaxis. There have been claims and
counterclaims, charges and countercharges. It would be
of great benefit to clear the air. Modern obstetrics has
set for itself the goal not only of a healthy mother and
baby, but also of a *happy* mother and baby. Let it be
stated once and for all that the first consideration—the
health and welfare of mother and child—is *never* subor-
dinated to the second. It has been charged that practi-

tioners of psychoprophylaxis place the "method" and its accomplishments first and will not utilize modern obstetrical knowledge and skills that might benefit a mother and child. This is simply not true. If a baby *must* be delivered by obstetrical forceps because of the nature of the labor, this is, of course, done. However, critics of prepared labor usually believe in the routine use of amnesia for labor, the routine incision of the vaginal opening (episiotomy), and the more or less routine use of obstetrical forceps and anesthesia. These techniques are used with a prepared mother only when they are necessary, not as a routine procedure.

The charge has been made that practitioners of prepared labor refuse to administer pain-relieving medications (analgesics) to women in labor because the "method" does not call for it; that women are permitted to suffer needlessly because medication that could afford relief is intentionally withheld. Again, critics of prepared labor claim that the woman is sacrificed to the "method." Nothing could be further from the truth. Analgesics can be and are easily and regularly administered in appropriate dosages to prepared mothers *if and when they are needed*. It is, however, the common experience of obstetricians that even when the prepared woman needs medication, she needs far less than the unprepared mother usually does. And it is unquestionable that the smaller the dosage, the better for the baby.

Many American women think that "natural childbirth" is "childbirth in the raw." They think that the use of analgesics must be entirely eliminated; that their use must not even be considered. It is these women who have been misled by the propaganda against prepared labor. They have seized upon the inaccurate word "natural" and made it their cause. They have created an approach in which they commit obstetrical suicide, sacrificing themselves on the altar of the method. This is the very thing psychoprophylaxis endeavors to avoid.

Psychoprophylaxis is goal-oriented—it hopes to provide a way to achieve delivery of a baby by a mother who is fully awake, completely aware, and actively participating in the birth of her child. All effort is expended toward the achievement of this goal. Psychoprophylaxis is *not* method-oriented. There are no medals for the proper execution of the exercise techniques, there are no diplomas for attendance at Prenatal Class, there are no examinations to pass. The only grades, medals, and diplomas lie within each mother and are awarded by her to herself for having accomplished what she set out to do. Success in prepared labor can be measured by the pleasure of the mothers and their eagerness to have their next child the same way. This is the only true test. It serves no useful purpose to ascertain how "natural" the labor and delivery were by measuring against some arbitrary standard, if the mother would reject a similar experience with her next confinement.

Now that we have discussed what psychoprophylaxis is, and what it is not, we will make a detailed examination of the biological and cultural aspects of human childbirth. Understanding childbirth is essential to understanding psychoprophylaxis. For those who will train in psychoprophylaxis in formal classes, the material presented here will supplement what they will learn in class. For those who will not attend classes, it will provide the necessary background for understanding the technique and using the training exercises, which are described later.

II

The Biology of Childbirth

The only constant thing about childbirth throughout all of human history has been its biology—the equipment provided men and women for reproduction and the functions performed by this equipment. Human reproduction is classified as viviparous; that is, the fully formed human child is born from the mother, not, for example, as a fertilized egg and then growing and developing outside of the mother as in oviparous reproduction.

The organs provided the woman to meet the requirements for viviparous reproduction are few and multipurpose. Within the abdomen lie two flat, corrugated glands, approximately $1 \times 1\frac{1}{2}$ inches in size, that contain the ova (egg cells). Not only do these ovaries contain the reproductive cells; they also manufacture hormones that are essential to the reproductive process. Also within the abdomen is the uterus (womb), a hollow, muscular bag that in the nonpregnant woman is about $3\frac{1}{2} \times 2 \times 1\frac{1}{2}$ inches in size. The uterus connects with the outside through its cervix (or neck) which juts into the vagina, and it connects with the ovaries by means of two tubes (oviducts) arising from the sides of its fundus (top). The tubes increase in diameter as they approach the ovaries, terminating in an umbrellalike end with many tiny fingerlike projections. When a mature ovum is ejected from the ovary (ovulation), the end of the tube envelops the ovary so that the egg is thrust into the interior of the tube. The egg can now be reached by spermatozoa from the father. When spermatozoa are deposited in the vagina during coitus (sexual intercourse) they come into contact with the cervix of the uterus. The ovarian hor-

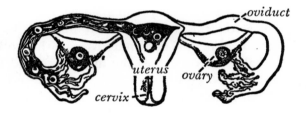

The passage of one fertilized ovum from ovary to implantation in the uterus.

mones mentioned before prepare the cervix to be most receptive to spermatozoa at ovulation time. Therefore, the spermatozoa traverse the cervix with ease, are transported through the uterine cavity and into the tubes. Here one of them comes into contact with the ovum and fertilizes it—and a new individual is conceived. Thus pregnancy is achieved.

The fertilized ovum is then slowly transported down the tube and into the uterine cavity. In the meantime, ovarian hormones have prepared the lining of the uterus, thickening it and causing its glands to excrete a sugar-rich substance to nourish it. On approximately the twenty-fifth day after the onset of the previous menstrual period, the ovum finds a suitable place in the fundus of the uterus, embeds itself within the uterine wall, covers itself with maternal tissue, and proceeds on its way to full development. The embryo surrounds itself with two membranes. The inner membrane is filled with fluid in which the baby floats. Part of the outer membrane develops into the placenta (afterbirth), the organ by which the developing child feeds and maintains itself. The baby connects to the placenta through its umbilical cord. The maternal side of the placenta consists of millions of microscopic projections that bathe in maternal blood. From this blood, across the membrane and into the baby's blood, come oxygen, food and vitamins from the mother. From the baby's blood, across the membrane and into the mother's blood go carbon dioxide and waste products. And thus, snug and secure, well shielded from the outside world, the baby develops and grows to maturity.

Delivery of the infant must be effected at the *appropriate time*. The phrase "appropriate time" cannot be overemphasized; it is miraculous that such an overwhelming percentage of infants are born healthy, quite mature, and ready for the rigors of the outside world. During the 264 days (more or less) of pregnancy, the uterus, cervix, and vagina undergo profound changes in preparation for the expected labor. The maternal mechanical problem is amazing. The conceptus and its surrounding membranes must be retained for 264 days in order to deliver a mature infant. The cervix must remain closed during this entire period, holding in, at term, about ten pounds in baby, fluid, and membranes. The uterus must remain quiescent during this period

of development and growth. Then at the appropriate
time, the uterus must contract in a manner that causes
the cervix to dilate slowly, without maternal damage,
permitting the infant to be thrust slowly forward through
the birth canal. Once through the cervix, the infant must
traverse the vagina. This structure must, therefore, be
capable of stretching markedly without tearing to accommodate the infant.

The entire process—the retention of the infant for the
proper time, the gradual opening of the cervix and expulsion of the infant—is usually completed with essentially no damage to the mother. As far as damage to the
infant is concerned, there are those who believe that in
normal instances, labor is actually beneficial to the infant—whether because of its stimulatory effects on the
infant or because of some unknown effect.

The ability of uterus, cervix, and vagina to fulfill their
assigned tasks during labor and delivery does not come
about by chance or good fortune. From the earliest days
of pregnancy changes occur in the cervix and vagina to
prepare them for labor and delivery. The blood supply
of the cervix increases markedly, causing a change in
color from the usual pink to blue or violet. The cervix
also becomes markedly softened, not only because of the
increased blood supply but also because of actual swelling. The glands that line the canal of the cervix become
more highly developed and join together into a "honeycomb" filled with mucus. This "mucus honeycomb" is
called the cervical mucus plug, and it effectively protects
the contents of the uterus from vaginal contamination.

The increased blood supply, swelling and softening
of the cervix permit it to accomplish its task during
labor. The cervix starts as a long, cylindrical structure,

but because of uterine contractions the cervix is "taken up" (before labor in first pregnancies; during labor, as a rule, in subsequent ones). It is converted from a cylindrical structure with openings to the uterus and the vagina to a conical structure that is continuous with the walls of the uterus, leaving only one opening between the uterine cavity and the vagina. A tough fibrous cervix could not readily undergo this change. (The process is called cervical effacement and is described according to how completely the cervix is effaced—complete effacement of the cervix is called "one hundred percent efface" and so on.)

The second demand placed upon the cervix is that it dilate, slowly but progressively, once again in response to uterine contractions. This permits the infant to move out of the uterus and into the vagina. Some dilatation may occur in response to contractions before labor, but most of the dilating is done during labor in both first and subsequent pregnancies. (The amount of dilatation is commonly expressed in centimeters or "fingers." Ten centimeters or five fingers constitute full dilatation of the cervix.)

The vagina undergoes changes as well. Its blood supply becomes richer, and like the cervix it changes from pink to violet blue. The vaginal lining thickens, and the supporting tissues surrounding the vagina loosen. The muscular elements contained within the vaginal wall increase in size, so that frequently there is an actual increase in vaginal length. This can result in slight protrusion of the vaginal wall through the external vaginal opening. It should be apparent that these changes prepare the vagina for the great degree of distention it must undergo during delivery. The tissues of the vaginal outlet—skin, muscles, and supporting elements—are similarly altered to permit easier distention. During pregnancy the vaginal secretion is considerably increased. It is highly acid and probably plays an important role in keeping the vagina relatively free of harmful bacteria.

Much mention has already been made of the functions of uterine contractions in labor. It can easily be imagined that these contractions must have considerable force in order to change the form of the cervix and to expel the infant. The muscle power required of uterine contractions is considerably greater than the nonpregnant uterus can generate. How does the uterine muscle acquire its reinforcements?

The nonpregnant uterus is a muscular bag roughly $3\frac{1}{2} \times 2 \times 1$ inches in size, as has been stated before. The growth during pregnancy is incredible: at term the uterus measures $15 \times 10 \times 8$ inches, an increase of some 520 times in capacity. The weight of the uterus increases as well, from a few ounces to about $2\frac{1}{4}$ pounds at term— thus the increase in uterine size does not represent merely the stretching of existing muscle fibers over the growing conceptus. The individual muscle fibers of which the uterus is composed increase markedly in both length and breadth. This increase in fiber size occurs partly because more actomyosin, the contractile protein, is deposited within the muscle fiber, permitting each fiber to exert more force. With most muscles this type of change is achieved through hard exercise. This is clearly impossible for uterine muscle, so actomyosin is provided without the stimulus of exercise. The uterus at term will have the contractile capability to do the work demanded of it during a normal birth.

We have already noted that the uterine muscle must

not use its great contractile potential until the appropriate time. Throughout pregnancy the uterus contracts in a disorganized and uncoordinated fashion, but an elaborate system prevents these contractions from affecting the pregnancy. The exact mechanism of this "uterine brake" is unknown. However, at the proper moment the "brake" is disengaged and regular and rhythmic contractions begin. They occur in a well-organized and well-coordinated fashion, each contraction carefully patterned to do the most work. The work of each contraction can be measured by its effect—progress in labor. (Progress in

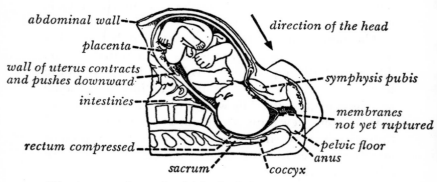

The passage through which the baby is born consists of the cervix (or outlet of the uterus) and the vagina (or birth canal). When labor begins the muscles of the uterus rhythmically contract and relax; they shorten a little each time, thus gradually thinning and pulling up the cervix. The first stage of labor is when these contractions open the cervix. The second stage is when the baby is being pushed out of the uterus through the open cervix and down the birth canal.

labor is, in turn, measured by the increasing dilatation of the cervix and the descent of the infant in the birth canal.) The normal spread of the contraction wave across the uterus in labor is from the top of the uterus (fundus) toward the cervix. This could not be more logical, for it results in the gradual application of the forces of labor in the one direction in which they must be exerted to achieve progress. It is a most remarkably designed system and unquestionably a most effective one.

The course of labor is divided, for descriptive purposes, into three stages. The first stage of labor begins with the onset of regular, progressive uterine contractions and ends when the cervix is completely dilated. The second stage of labor begins when the cervix is fully dilated and ends when the infant is delivered. The third stage of labor begins when the infant is delivered and ends when the placenta (afterbirth) is delivered.

During the first stage, the uterus contracts and causes the cervix to dilate. The contractions at the beginning of labor are usually rather infrequent and of short duration and low intensity. As labor progresses, the contractions increase in frequency, intensity, and duration. This increase occurs slowly and deliberately throughout the first stage, reaching its height when there are from seven to ten centimeters of cervical dilatation (called the transitional first stage). Contractions now would be occurring about every two minutes, lasting about fifty to sixty seconds and of strong intensity. This frequency and duration are rarely exceeded.

With full dilatation of the cervix, the intensity of the contractions diminishes somewhat. There is, as a rule, greater comfort, perhaps because the cervix is no longer an obstacle and the conceptus is no longer forced against it with each contraction. Now, for the first time, forces other than the contraction of the uterus itself must be exerted. Voluntary expulsive efforts (pushing) at each

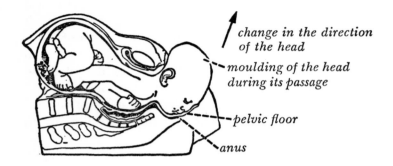

change in the direction
of the head

moulding of the head
during its passage

pelvic floor

anus

Until the baby's head passes under the symphysis pubis (the cartilage that joins the two pelvic bones) it slips back a little after each contraction. By this time the membranes have broken. With each contraction the doctor can see more and more of the forehead and nose. Note how the baby has turned so that he faces toward his mother's back.

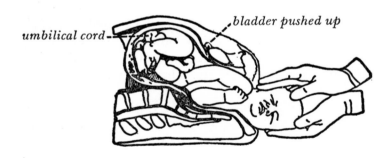

umbilical cord

bladder pushed up

Soon the shoulders emerge. The doctor's hands support and guide the baby's head and shoulders as he is born.

contraction, if properly done, are quite effective in propelling the infant through the remainder of the birth canal.

The third stage of labor, separation and delivery of the placenta, is usually accomplished without problems or difficulties. The placenta separates from the uterine wall with three or four postdelivery contractions and is expelled, in most instances, with minimal maternal effort. However, separation of the placenta leaves large open blood vessels in the uterine wall. Uterine contraction closes them but until this can be effected, there is bleeding. It is therefore normal to lose a glass to a glass and a half (250 to 400 cc.) of blood after delivery. This is to be expected, not feared.

Voluntary muscles (so-called skeletal muscles), such as those of the arms and legs, are more or less completely dominated by the higher centers of the brain and respond only to *consciously* given instructions from the brain. However, the muscle of which the uterus is composed is smooth or involuntary muscle, like the muscle of the intestines or urinary bladder. This type of muscle contracts independent of the will. Therefore the functions of the pregnant uterus and the mechanisms controlling and coordinating its activity are not under conscious, volitional control. The "uterine brake" previously described is applied and disengaged independent of the will. Once labor is started, it continues independent of the will. One cannot will the onset of labor, nor can one consciously and deliberately alter the pattern of labor once it begins. It proceeds inexorably to its termination regardless of the desires of the woman in whom it happens to be occurring.

This, then, is childbirth. It is the phenomenon that

ends a 264-day process, all of the phases of which are integrated toward one end—delivery of a healthy, mature child with minimal effect to mother and baby. It should be abundantly clear how beautifully this objective is reached. In a biological sense, it has been reached the same way since the first woman walked the earth. But what human civilization has done with this magnificent biology is quite another matter. The current obstetrical dilemma in America did not just happen. It is part of a long and fascinating story, which begins with the first humans. Let us, therefore, begin at the beginning.

III

The Early History of Childbirth

"And the Lord God said unto the woman: 'What is this thou has done?' And the woman said: 'The serpent beguiled me, and I did eat.' And the Lord God said unto the serpent: 'Because thou has done this, cursed art thou from among all cattle, and from among all beasts of the field; upon thy belly shalt thou go, and dust shalt thou eat all the days of thy life. And I will put enmity between thee and the woman, and between thy seed and her seed; they shall bruise thy head, and thou shalt bruise their heel.' Unto the woman He said: 'I will greatly multiply thy pain and thy travail; in pain thou shalt bring forth children; and thy desire shall be to thy husband, and he shall rule over thee.' " [1]

And so it began, because of an apple.

On the island of Borneo, there is a legend about the origin of midwifery. Kelili went into the jungle with his wife Teburi, who was pregnant. As he went along, look-

[1] Hertz, J. H., translator, *The Pentateuch and Haftorahs*, Vol. 1, pp. 10–12.

ing for food, he came to the place of the big monkeys. He then saw what he had never seen before. A young pregnant female was calling out in pain. She crouched, and her mate waited beside her until the birth was over. Kelili waited and watched and learned his lesson. He had seen how the husbands among the big monkeys help their wives at the delivery of their young. And so when his own Teburi went into labor, he helped her throughout, as he had seen the monkey husband doing.

This is the story of one primitive people; other peoples and regions have their own. How accurately these legends, as retold in modern times, represent the real beginnings of tribal customs is difficult to say. But birth attendance was introduced into human culture very early, and it is probable that as in the legend from Borneo, the first birth attendants were the husbands. One might speculate that this was so because these peoples lived somewhat isolated from one another, in family units, and the husband may have been the only other adult available. It is known that the most primitive people did not connect childbearing with sexual relations, so the husband was not chosen because of his responsibility for the pregnancy. It is rather more likely that he was chosen simply because he was there.

How did this husband attend his wife—what did he offer her in the way of assistance? Realistically speaking, he probably offered her little technical assistance. But he did give her comfort, companionship, and solace at the time of her travail. And it is this that must be hailed as the first great contribution. How different to have someone close by, to know that one is not alone! Needless to say childbirth at this time was a rather hazardous undertaking. Even though the woman might be in excellent physical condition, there was absolutely no way to cope with the abnormal birth. It is likely, therefore, that not only did many babies succumb, but many mothers as well. Since human beings can transmit experience to others and to their own offspring, it is certain that our primitive mother-to-be knew of the hazards. How much nicer, therefore, to have one's mate at one's side.

Behavior often, particularly in primitive societies, tends to become stylized and ritualistic. Thus once fathers had begun to attend births it was inevitable that they would develop some standard behavior. A primitive father, in attending his wife, may, for example, have sat behind her and then to the right. As all went well, he tended to sit in the same position the next time. As such patterns were repeated, the husband gradually assumed a more complicated role in the childbirth complex. He even became an early midwife, sitting behind his wife and pressing on her abdomen with contractions. He also became the first nurse and pediatrician, attending the newborn, severing the cord by cutting or biting, and then cleaning or painting the child.

Thus from a mere companion the father became an important part of a stylized, culturally determined behavior complex. Then as now, childbirth was cultural, not "natural"; women approached labor conditioned to expect certain experiences, and they reacted to these experiences in the manner prescribed by the rituals and traditions of their culture and society. The history of childbirth customs from this point on is merely a record of changing patterns and attitudes and of the effects of scientific advances.

One of the strangest birth customs, the couvade, arose in widely divergent areas of the world, apparently spontaneously. The husband, formerly an active integral participant in the birth, instead assumed a passive symbolic role: At or before the birth of the child, the father behaved as if he and not his wife were being confined. This ritual, which still exists in some parts of the world, may assume many forms. The husband may go to bed and groan and writhe to indicate the pain he endures. Couvade may merely represent a belief that the pregnancy suffers if the husband is injured—for example, a miscarriage may be attributed to a fall by the husband.

How did this most peculiar practice arise? The answer will probably never be known. Some feel that it stems from the time in history when both sexes gave milk. Others have suggested that it represents the concept of original sin, placing equal burden upon the man. However it arose, it seems to constitute in some cultures the transition from the custom of expecting the husband to assist at his wife's labor to the custom of entirely excluding the husband from the confinement.

As a culture became more complex, its childbirth rituals and practices also became more complex. Childbirth in many cultures became a purely female venture, with the husband and other men completely excluded. The women chosen to assist were almost always older women who were ostensibly experienced in childbirth, at least from having themselves given birth. It is possible that this change again represented a practical step forward, an advance in social organization as family units became less isolated and developed a community life on a tribal basis. Within a social structure where there is a common sense of interdependence, the pregnant woman can seek and receive aid from outside her immediate family unit. It did not, of course, follow that this change brought with it improvement in the quality of the care rendered. Childbirth continued to be beset with ritual, magic, and superstition. Among the Maoris of New Zealand, for instance, there was a strict order of precedence among birth assistants: the maternal grandmother, then the paternal grandmother, and finally the mother-in-law, regardless of their qualifications.

The employment of "wise women" from without the family was a later development. These were the primitive midwives, the first professional birth attendants. In some tribes, arrangements were made well in advance for the services of such a woman at a birth, and it became customary to reward her with gifts, and later on with formal payment. Eventually a woman could be well attended, probably in her own home, by anywhere from one to several "wise women." It is doubtful if these women did more than press upon her abdomen with the contractions and attend to the cord and child. No doubt they had their charms, incantations, amulets, and rituals. But merely by constant observation of the birth process, they inevitably acquired a larger fund of objective knowledge than had ever been accumulated before. This they were able to pass on to others, and so slowly arose the truly professional, trained midwife, in possession of all the subjective and objective information available at the time.

Such midwives were occasionally consulted during pregnancy, usually about the sex of the child. Mexican midwives began kneading the abdomen daily from the seventh month on to prevent abnormal presentations of the baby. If the abnormal position persisted, the woman was turned upside down and violently shaken. As a rule these midwives confined their care to the labor and delivery, though in some areas they rendered care into the puerperium (period following birth) as well. Not all of the care they rendered was good. Among desert tribes in Algeria, for example, the midwife would delay the birth of the child for fifteen minutes by firmly holding the head after it emerged and preventing the remainder of the child from being delivered. Swahili midwives singed the pubic hairs before labor to remove demons that might be lurking there.

This kind of obstetrical practice worked well in an overwhelming number of normal cases. But what of the abnormal? There were as yet no male or physician midwives. Abnormal births were regarded as the work of demons, and powerful demons required the shaman. Labor was considered a voluntary act by the child desirous of escaping from the uterus. Thus if labor did not proceed well the child was coaxed with food or even threatened. Attempts might be made to frighten the child out of the womb. Failing in these efforts, it then became logical to force the child out by exerting various forms of pressure on the abdomen with straps, blows, and so on. If the midwives still could not effect delivery, they might turn to men who were shepherds or swineherds. These men would apply the experience gained with their flocks and would extract the child piece by piece from the uterus.

The obstetrical practice of midwives as developed by primitive tribes remained essentially unchanged for many centuries. The rise of the priest-physician and later the physician who was not a priest made available to the midwives, for the first time, a trained healer who was skilled in the medicine and surgery of his day. Now when delivery could not be effected, the physician was called. The *Sushruta Samhita,* an Indian text dating from the 4th century A.D., says that delivery should be conducted by four midwives "stouthearted and of ripe age, who shall trim their nails well." A doctor was consulted in any unusual case, and the text describes in detail what to do in any contingency. Many of the techniques described are still practiced today. Since the Indian physician was also a priest, his duties extended past the delivery. Breast feeding could begin only with his approval. He had to be present at the first feeding to deliver this incantation: "May four oceans, full of milk, constantly abide in both your breasts, you blessed one, for the increase of the strength of the child. Drinking of the milk, whose sap is the sap of immortal life divine, may your boy gain long life, as do the gods by feeding on the beverage of immortality." [2]

A similar type of obstetrical practice existed in ancient Persia, Israel, and Egypt. Knowledge was meager, professional skill was lacking, superstition was great. But the mother was well cared for. Women were actively attended in their own homes, except for those of high caste, who went to a "birth house" to deliver.

With the emergence of great schools of medicine in Greece, a foundation was laid for medical practice based upon sound observation and reasoned conclusion. However, there was little advancement in obstetrical knowledge and skill, because childbirth remained the province of the midwives. Hippocrates and his followers were called to attend births only to effect deliveries when the midwives failed. Since they had no experience with normal labors, they learned little. Hippocrates mentions little of obstetrics in his voluminous writings, and much

[2] Graham, H., *Eternal Eve,* p. 30.

of what he does say is misinformation. In *The Nature of the Infant* he states, "Among women in labor, those who suffer most are the primiparae [women delivering their first child], because they have not previously experienced this kind of suffering. They suffer in the whole body, but especially in the lumbar region and ischia; for their ischia separate." [3] Thus for centuries it was believed that the pelvic bones separate to make room for the baby, and the idea of a disproportion between the infant's head and mother's pelvis was not entertained. Hippocrates also supported the commonly held concept of his era that the infant initiates labor and that the forces of labor are fetal forces.

The Greek women delivered at home, with their husbands at their sides. They used special obstetrical chairs that took advantage of the force of gravity and permitted the midwives to assist the birth. There was usually a chief midwife and several assistants. Greek midwives were required to be mothers themselves and to be past the age of childbearing. Perhaps they had all the training available in Athens in 400 B.C. One of their most important functions was advising young men on the potential fertility of maidens. They thus became the most important matchmakers and achieved considerable influence. [4]

The civilizations of Rome, Byzantium, and the Dark Ages and Middle Ages of Europe made few advancements in the obstetrical art and science. Women were attended in more or less the same fashion for fifteen centuries. The normal birth was no problem and was well conducted and attended by midwives. Obstructed labors and faulty presentations of the infant presented prob-

[3] Graham, *op. cit.,* p. 49.
[4] Graham, *op. cit.*

lems beyond the ability of either the midwives or the physicians. Caesarean section was known, but since such surgery was entirely unsafe, it meant an attempt to save the child at the expense of the mother. The other solution was to extract the child piecemeal—thus saving the mother at the expense of the child. There were other procedures, but they tended to sacrifice both mother and child. It was not until the sixteenth and seventeenth centuries that techniques were developed to achieve the delivery of a living infant from a living mother. The most important of these techniques was "the secret of the Chamberlens," which will be described in the next chapter.

IV

Science Enters Childbirth

Obstetrics, like many other fields of learning, changed greatly during the Renaissance. The introduction of the printing press permitted the wide distribution of medical textbooks; the Germans, with characteristic organizational zeal, began to regulate the instruction and qualifications of midwives. But neither regulation nor textbooks could solve the problem of the obstructed birth, and certain obstetrical complications, such as hemorrhage and severe infection, were impossible to treat and invariably resulted in maternal death. Knowledge of the nature of blood and its circulation was inadequate at best, and Pasteur had yet to be born.

Soranus of Ephesus, who practiced in Rome about 100 A.D., had been the first to describe a procedure for delivering a child by grasping its feet while still in the uterus, turning it around, and effecting delivery by pulling gently on the feet. Soranus, a great proponent of rational midwifery, attempted to discourage superstition and the use of brute force. His work, however, was lost, and it was not until 1551 that the procedure was again described, this time by the great Ambroise Paré. Paré was the greatest surgeon of his day. The fact that he was interested in and practiced obstetrics did a great deal to establish the prestige and respectability of the field and to rekindle interest in it among physicians.

In his first obstetrical writings, Paré described the method of podalic version. He did not claim that he invented the method but rather that he had seen others in Paris practicing it. He wrote: "And supposing that the child presents naturally having the head towards the outlet, to duly deliver it by art, you must gently push it back in the contrary direction and seek the feet and draw them down. By doing this you will easily turn the child. And when you have drawn the feet into the outlet you must draw one foot outside and tie it above the heel in the manner of a running noose with a moderately long fillet, like that with which women bind their hair. Then you will replace the said foot into the said womb and having found the other foot you will draw it outside and then pull on the fillet, and when you have thus both feet outside the womb you will draw on both equally on one side as on the other, little by little and without violence." [5] The midwives were to assist with the delivery of the aftercoming head.

It was no longer necessary to leave the mother with an obstructed labor to languish without a chance or sacrifice either mother or child. An attempt could be made to deliver her of a live baby. This difference in approach cannot be emphasized too strongly, for it has become the cornerstone of modern obstetrics: to deliver a live and healthy mother of a live and healthy baby.

[5] Graham, *op. cit.*, p. 152.

Late in the sixteenth century the Chamberlen brothers, Peter the Elder and Peter the Younger, became
famous as barber-surgeons and especially as practitioners
of obstetrics. Peter the Elder became physician to King
James I and his Queen Anne. Both brothers developed
reputations for being able to deliver women where all
others had failed. How they achieved this no one knew,
for they kept the method to themselves. When called
upon to deliver a woman, they would arrive at the home
in a special carriage. They entered the lying-in chamber
carrying a huge wooden box decorated with gilded carv-
ings—always carried by the two of them. The mother was
blindfolded, and everyone except the Chamberlens was
excluded from the room. The door was then locked.
Peculiar noises, ringing bells, sinister sounds of all sorts
emanated from the room as they put their secret to work.
When the baby was delivered, the secret was replaced in
the large wooden box and the lid was locked, and only
then were the doors opened.

What was this secret that the Chamberlens possesssed?
Being barber-surgeons, they were maligned both by the
College of Physicians (admittance was by M.D. degree
only) and by the midwives. But no one could argue with
success, and they were continually being called in for
consultation by the midwives.

Not only did the brothers Chamberlen have a secret,
but they had a vigorous social conscience as well. They
championed the formation of a society of midwives and
formal instruction and examination for midwives. This
placed them in direct opposition to the College of Physicians. Interestingly enough, the only supervision of midwifery at that time was carried on by the Church, which

was interested in childbirth for two reasons: to encourage baptism of the babies, and to discourage the use of heathen charms, amulets, or incantations. Thus the campaign of the two Peters also put them in opposition to the Church. They filed a petition with the College of Physicians advocating their cause. The College promptly adopted a resolution prohibiting a society of midwives and rejected the proposal for regulated instruction and examination.

Peter the Younger married and had eight children. The eldest child, another Peter, received the degree of Doctor of Medicine (which neither his father nor his uncle possessed) in 1619 and was therefore admitted to fellowship in the College of Physicians. He was a brilliant young man and soon became the best male midwife in the land, possessing and using the secret of the Chamberlens. He also took up the campaign of his father and uncle to organize and license midwives.

The secret was passed through two more generations of Chamberlens. In the early years of the eighteenth century, forceps used for the delivery of live babies from live mothers came into common use. Their origin was frequently attributed to the Chamberlens. But it was not until 1813 that their mysterious methods were finally made known. A box was discovered in the attic of the last Dr. Chamberlen after his death. It contained, among other things, three pairs of obstetrical forceps. The three sets of forceps showed progressive improvement in design and were probably the ones used by Peter I, II, and III respectively. They were straight, with fenestrated blades and rounded edges so as not to injure the child's head. This, then, was the

great secret—the obstetrical forcep, the first instrument
that could deliver a living baby from a living mother in
obstructed labors.

Thus there occurred a minor revolution in obstetrical
care. With podalic version and forceps, two excellent
methods of dealing with problem labors were available,
and male midwives began to come into their own. Coin-
cidentally, greater interest arose in the instruction and
regulation of midwives. The entire birth process came
under greater scrutiny. Investigations in anatomy were
becoming more numerous, and more accurate information about the internal organs of reproduction was dis-
seminated. Through all of this scientific revolution, the
comfort and welfare of the individual mother-to-be was
foremost in the minds of her attendants. The vast majority delivered at home in their own beds, surrounded by
their families, midwives and obstetricians. All assistance
and examinations were performed by the physician with
the privie parts covered, for it was unseemly that a man
should see these.

As occurs in the usual course of human events, the
inevitable squabble over who should conduct the labor
and deliver the baby arose. Were the midwives to offi-
ciate until the physician was needed? Was the physician
to take charge, with the midwives acting under him?
In Laurence Sterne's novel *Tristram Shandy,* first published in 1760, the narrator's mother, Mrs. Shandy, comes
to grips with this problem. Since she is to be confined
at the country house, she must do without the attentions
of Sir Richard Manningham. Her choice is, therefore, an
experienced midwife, "notwithstanding there was a scientific operator within so near a call as eight miles of us,
and who, moreover, had expressly wrote a five-shillings

book upon the subject of midwifery." Mr. Shandy finally agreed to the midwife, but only if Dr. Slop, the "scientific operator," was in attendance as well. "In a word, my mother was to have the old woman and the operator was to have license to drink a bottle of wine with my father and my Uncle Toby Shandy in the back parlour, for which he was to be paid five guineas."

Slowly, of course, the situation began to resolve itself, with the doctors becoming more and more popular. Many books on the subject were written and criticized, and as doctors gathered more experience, the books became more accurate. The idea of lying-in hospitals was advanced and accepted. It must be remembered that science—exact observation—had by this time pervaded the medical profession. Autopsy was common and in some hospitals compulsory.

The largest lying-in hospital of the late eighteenth century was at the Allegemeines Krankenhaus in Vienna. The first professor of midwifery and director of the hospital was Dr. Lucas Johann Boer. He served the institution with distinction for thirty-four years, then was forced to retire because his enemies thought he was getting too old and conservative. Dr. Boer taught midwifery on a mannequin, refusing to use female cadavers. During his tenure, the annual mortality of mothers from all causes was 1.3%. In 1822 he was replaced by his assistant, Johann Klein.

Now things went modern. The mannequins were discarded, and instruction was given directly on female cadavers. From the autopsy room the new scientists went directly to the bedside. The maternal mortality rate of 1.3% rose dramatically to 7.8% in Klein's first year. Nor was this the only setback for the new methods. In 1840 the maternity service of the hospital was divided into two clinics, the first for the instruction of medical students, the second for the instruction of midwives. In the first clinic, medical students were instructed on the cadaver, performed dissections, and were encouraged to examine their patients frequently. The midwives of the second clinic, on the other hand, had no such good fortune. They were instructed upon the mannequin only and were not even allowed in the dissecting rooms. Needless to say, their examinations of patients were limited to what they could see and what they could feel through the belly. Internal examinations were beyond their scope. By 1846 the maternal mortality rate in the first clinic was four times that of the second clinic. This became well known among the pregnant women, many of whom refused to be delivered in the first clinic, pleading to be allowed to die at home or be delivered by the midwives of the second clinic.

The forces of history have a way of providing the man for the job, once the requirements of the job have been defined. In 1846, Ignaz Philipp Semmelweis, a Hungarian, assumed the duties of assistant to Dr. Klein in the first clinic. By this time the previously low mortality rates had been forgotten, and the 9.9% death rate in the first clinic was accepted as normal by all—except Semmelweis. He immediately set out to determine the cause. He first proceeded to examine and demolish all the theories advanced through that time, because they applied equally to both clinics. Semmelweis then proceeded to make two fundamental observations. First, that deaths from "childbed fever" were more common in women with long, tedious labors—twenty-four to forty-eight hours. Second, that women who delivered at home or on their way to the hospital rarely contracted the disease. Half of these women were assigned to the first clinic and half to the second clinic, and here the incidence of childbed fever was the same.

It happened that Semmelweis' friend Professor Jakob Kolletschka sustained a small puncture wound of the finger while conducting an autopsy with his students. The knife that inflicted the wound was contaminated with infected material from the cadaver. Kolletschka then developed a disease, from which he died, which resembled childbed fever in its development and course. This resemblance struck Semmelweis, and he now made the final observation. Kolletschka died from fever resulting from a wound inflicted by a knife contaminated with cadaveric material. After childbirth a woman has an even greater wound at the site of the separation of the placenta from the uterus. The students carried infected material from the dissecting rooms to the labor and delivery facilities. They infected the women, who then developed childbed fever and died. Since the midwives of the second clinic did not attend or perform the dissections or perform internal examinations, they did not infect their patients. Hence the difference in mortality rates between the two clinics.

In 1847, Semmelweis introduced his solution. His students were instructed to scrub their hands thoroughly in chloride of lime before they had anything to do with the pregnant women. The death rate dropped precipitously—from 11.4% in 1846 to 1.27% in 1848. (The midwives had 1.33% that year.) With the evidence now in, Semmelweis wrote, "Decomposed animal organic material was conveyed by the examining finger, the operating hand, the bedclothes, the atmospheric air, sponges, and the hands of midwives and nurses, which come into contact with the genitals of women in labor or just confined; in a word, the carrier of the decomposed animal organic material is everything which can be rendered unclean by such material and then come into contact with the genitals of the patient." [6]

Needless to say, this brilliant theory was met with something less than enthusiasm throughout Europe. The great professors could not easily accept an explanation that made them the transmitters of a fatal disease. Semmelweis and his theory were ridiculed at every turn. But, slowly, his recommendations were put into effect. England was one of the first nations in which marked improvement in death rates was attained through the use of chlorine disinfection. Carl Braun of Vienna recognized this difference between English and Continental mortality rates, but attributed it to the fact that only married women were admitted to British hospitals, while only unmarried women were admitted to German and French hospitals. Semmelweis answered: "The reasons for the better results in England we have fully explained, but we never imagined that our prophylaxis was defective because we did not prescribe marriage as a protection against puerperal fever." [7]

The complete vindication of Semmelweis' theory came after his death. The existence of bacteria was first demonstrated in 1863. In 1879, Pasteur and his students established the causal relationship between childbed fever and the bacteria found in the uterine discharge after delivery.

The triumph of Semmelweis and the secret of the

[6] Graham, *op. cit.,* p. 411.
[7] Graham, *op. cit.,* p. 415.

Chamberlens were two of the three developments necessary to transport childbirth from the home to the hospital. In the United States the third development, anesthesia, was first used during childbirth in the same year that Semmelweis discovered how to prevent childbed fever—1847. Laughing gas, or nitrous oxide, had been discovered in 1772 by Joseph Priestley. It was used sporadically for dental procedures, but its effect was variable and it fell into disrepute. Ether had been known for many years, and in 1818, Michael Faraday, a student of Humphry Davy, noted that ". . . the vapor of ether mixed with common air . . . produces effects very similar to those occasioned by nitrous oxide." This observation was unknown in America, but by 1846, four men in this country had administered ether as an anesthetic agent. Finally, in 1847, Dr. Crawford W. Long of Jefferson, Georgia, used ether in his practice of midwifery, administering some to his wife at her confinement in 1847.

In England, the greatest obstetrician of his day, James Young Simpson, began to use ether in his practice sometime in 1846. However, the disadvantages of the agent prompted him to search for something more agreeable. After trying numerous liquids and chemicals, chloroform was suggested to Simpson. He introduced it into his practice, and its use soon became widespread.

As could be expected, the objections—both medical and moral—came in hot and heavy. Dublin obstetricians suggested that the use of chloroform would increase many of the complications of childbirth. Simpson promptly collected statistics to prove them wrong.

Clergymen argued against chloroform as a thwarting of the intent of God, as contrary to the Scriptures, as preventing the natural relationship to develop between mother and child by removing the suffering from childbirth. Simpson, of course, answered each of these arguments in turn.

The entire question was resolved for everyone in April 1853. Queen Victoria gave birth to Prince Leopold and was attended by Sir James Clark and Dr. John Snow, who administered chloroform to her. The queen was quite pleased with the effect. Needless to say, this resolved the issue, and anesthesia in childbirth was here to stay.

Before the introduction of anesthesia, childbirth still took place in the home, with midwives still primarily in attendance, and only a few women were delivered by physicians. The introduction of effective anesthesia, however, slowly altered this situation, since midwives could not use these agents, more and more doctors were to be found in the lying-in chamber. He could offer a woman relief of pain through anesthesia. If she were unable to deliver her baby for various reasons, he could apply his forceps. He now knew enough to wash his hands before attending to his patient, so that he himself no longer menaced her well-being.

During the succeeding years of the nineteenth century, there were no dramatic advances in obstetrical care. In 1902, however, the next important contribution was made. Chloroform could relieve the discomfort of the delivery. "Twilight sleep" could obliterate the labor as well. As originally introduced in Germany in 1902, morphine and scopolamine were given in combination, producing a dreamy half waking, half sleeping state and almost totally obliterating memory. Here, then, was the possibility of having a baby without knowing it. The

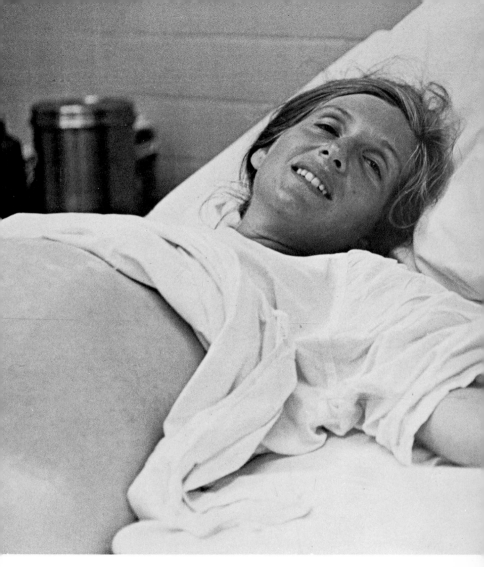

Mother in first stage of labor relaxes between contractions.

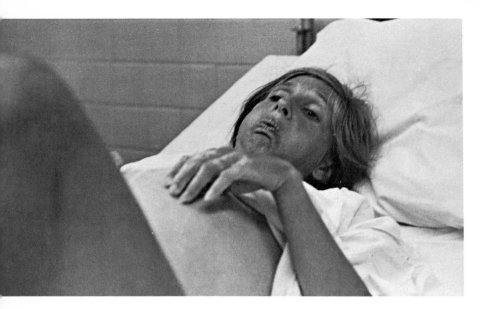

Now at the transitional stage, she uses the transitional breathing and effleurage (abdominal massage).

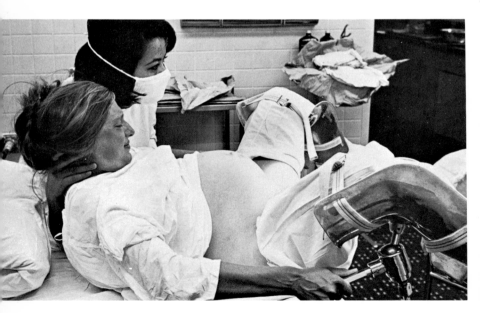

Moved into the delivery room, she pushes with second stage contractions.

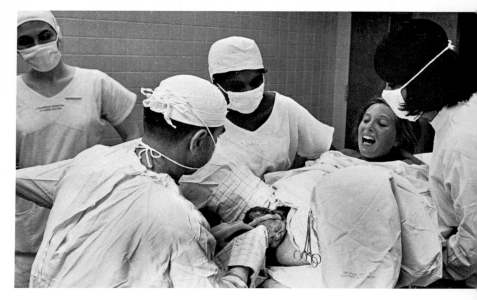

*Infant's head is born, and doctor removes one loop
of the umbilical cord from around it.*

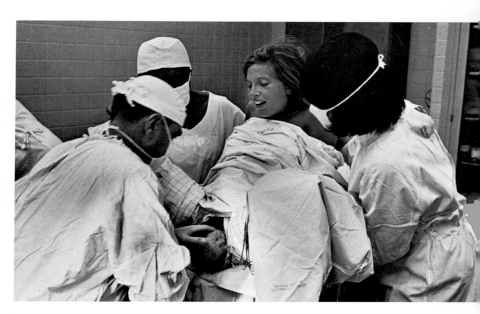

*Mother sits up to meet her child. Obstetrician applies gentle
downward pressure to effect delivery of upper shoulder.*

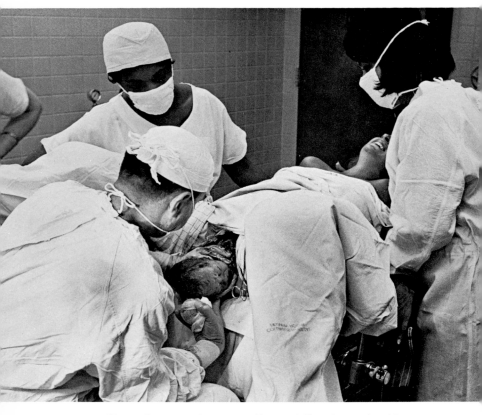

Upward pressure is now applied to deliver lower shoulder.

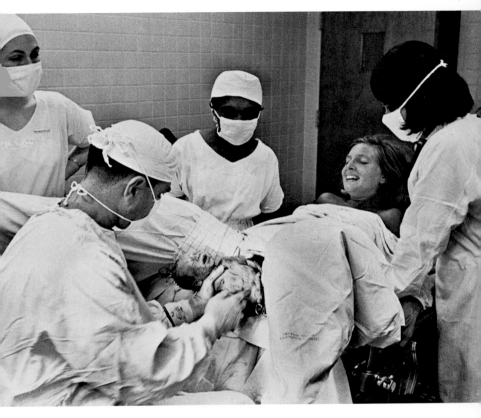

The infant has now begun to cry.

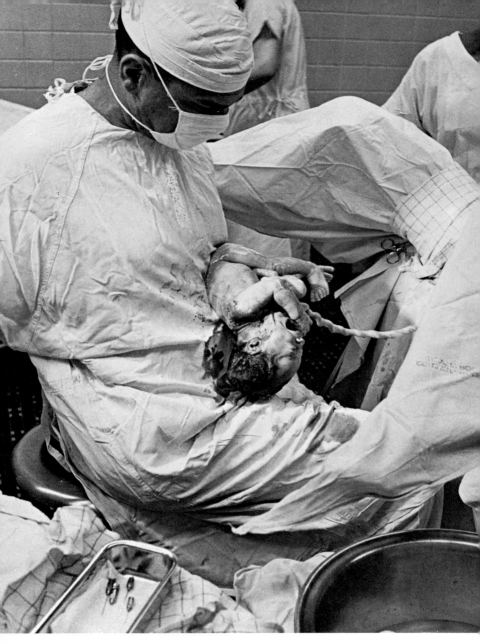

Infant is held head down after birth to assist drainage
of mucus from the respiratory passages.

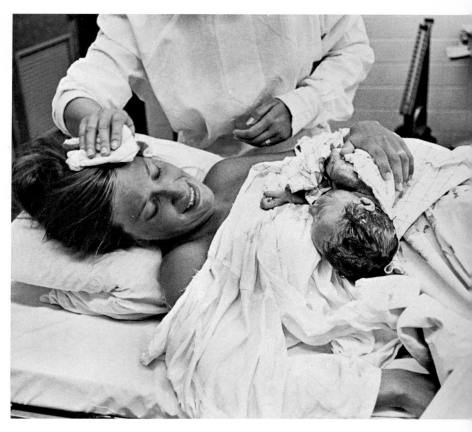

The cord has been cut, and mother meets her son.

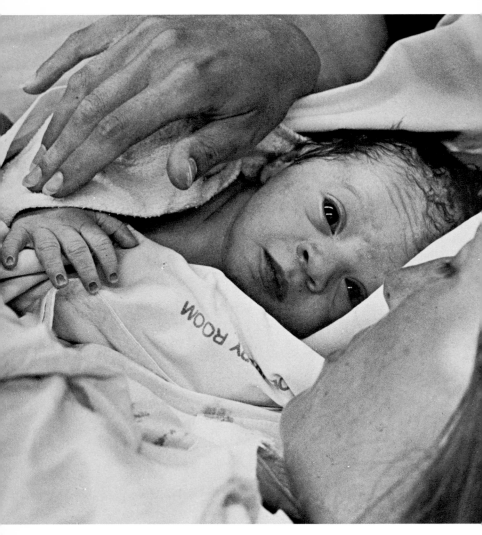

Minutes after birth . . .

method became rather popular in most quarters of the world, especially in the United States, where it was eagerly accepted by mothers-to-be. Since this method made it somewhat more difficult for a woman to deliver her baby with her own forces, and since it required a physician to administer drugs, the obstetrician became even more prominent in the United States. This kind of childbirth also encouraged the shift of scene from lying-in chamber in the home, surrounded by family and friends, to lying-in hospital, surrounded by twilight sleep. The lying-in hospital had previously been primarily the haven of the poor; others had their babies respectably at home. Now, however, the lying-in hospital slowly became the standard theater for the childbirth drama.

None of this could have happened if American society had not been ready to accept changes in its old ways and mores. In England it had taken Queen Victoria to get chloroform accepted. In the United States, however, the social climate was somewhat different. In the mid-nineteenth century there had begun a concerted drive to achieve civil equality for women. A "Declaration of Sentiments" was published in 1848 and reads in part: "The history of mankind is a history of repeated injuries and usurpations on the part of man toward woman, having in direct object the establishment of an absolute tyranny over her. . . . He has withheld from her rights which are given to the most ignorant and degraded men—both natives and foreigners. . . . women do feel themselves aggrieved, oppressed, and fraudulently deprived of their most sacred rights . . ." [8] Into this boiling pot of female discontent came the liberation from the one form of

[8] Johnson, C. O., *Government in the United States*, pp. 163-4.

"tyranny" with which the men had nothing to do—
childbirth. How eagerly these suffragettes must have
breathed in the chloroform, and later on how quickly
they accepted the injections of twilight sleep.

These ladies, clamoring as they were for equality with
men, could easily forfeit their "rights" in childbirth and
abdicate their role in the one *exclusive* female endeavor.
By the time twilight sleep had been introduced and
shown to be safe, the drive for women's rights had
reached its zenith. The success of women during the
First World War in replacing at home the men gone
off to war reinforced their desire to abdicate the role of
deliverers of children.

Had chloroform and twilight sleep come into the
world at a different time, it is doubtful if women would
have accepted them so readily. In their eagerness to liberate themselves from civil and social oppression, women
easily accepted what they considered liberation from
their biological oppression. For it was their biological
differences from men that made them women, and these
differences were at the bottom of the arguments used by
the male opponents of woman suffrage. One wonders if
women would have fought the powerful moral objections of the churches, particularly of the fundamentalist
Protestant churches prevalent in this country, if they had
already won the vote. Perhaps they would have chosen to
experience their biological destiny if they had already
achieved what they considered to be their social, politi-
cal and economic destiny.

V

Modern Obstetrics

The great scientific advances of the nineteenth and early twentieth centuries, which brought about the change of scene from home to hospital, also forced an unfortunate change in attitude toward the birth process itself. Formerly, birth was associated with the company of friends and normal health—despite the dangers. However, the modern era found birth associated with the hospital, the doctor, and illness—despite the increased safety.

How did a woman have a baby in the heyday of the midwife in the United States? She became pregnant and probably consulted the local midwife or physician in the later months of her pregnancy to arrange to be delivered. When she went into labor, her attendant was summoned and came to her home. She was usually surrounded by her husband, a friend or two, and the midwife and usually a doctor.

One obstetrician's advice, published in 1867, reads: "Before entering the room our arrival should always be announced; that we may not shock our patient by our unexpected entrance. We should take especial care to be ourselves in a happy frame of mind that we may appear in an easy, unaffected manner. And we should have no other thought in our mind than to attend strictly to our business in as agreeable a manner as possible." The doctor goes on to discuss the attendants: "The last rule to observe in relation to attendants is to have only the husband, the nurse, and the doctor. The husband at all events, and not more than two female friends; the doctor to be in and out from time to time, as his judgment may dictate. It is better to be absent as much as possible and keep due surveillance over the case, till toward the close of labor. In the first stage the female may make herself as comfortable as best she can, by walking about, sitting in her chair, or changing from one to the other. Unless the labor be very protracted, cold water is the only refreshment." [9]

This describes the fashion in which labors were conducted. Chloroform was now available for the delivery. Thus where there was a physician in attendance, this could be and was given. There was in all of this a certain dignity—the parturient woman was at the center of the stage, surrounded by loved ones and professional attendants as she brought her child into the world. The risks of childbirth were decreasing by now. Hemorrhage remained a problem, but obstructed labor, the demon of yesteryear, was yielding to the surgery made possible by chloroform and other anesthetics, and infection had been minimized by Semmelweis, soap, and water. But childbirth remained an essentially warm, close familial experience.

[9] Guernsey, H. N., *Obstetrics,* pp. 485, 488.

As medical and surgical techniques increased in complexity and variety, it became foolhardy to remain at home. The scene of the delivery had to be changed to the hospital. Once this change of scene was accomplished, however, the healthy childbirth, as well as the difficult childbirth, took place in the aseptic halls dedicated to the sick. The healthy young mother-to-be fell into the character of "patient" and began to be treated as such. She was registered, given a number. Her clothes and family were then taken away from her. Having no understanding of what she was undergoing or of what she was yet to undergo, she was put in a "labor room," either alone or with someone in similar straits, to labor. Deprived of the support of her husband and loved ones, placed in strange surroundings and left to her own devices, it was inevitable that she should be afraid. When faced with the choice of consciousness coupled with fear and pain or total oblivion, she naturally preferred oblivion. Under this new asepsis, maternity "patients" gleefully accepted medicated amnesia, labored, delivered, and woke to be told that they were mothers. It must be remembered, however, that this could never have come about if women had not been willing to *have* it happen.

Through all of this change, the first victim was the midwife. When pregnant women became "patients" there was no longer a need for her services, and she went the way of the horse, the blacksmith, and the carriage maker. The physician was the birth attendant. He was the only one who could legally create twilight sleep, and so he was in great demand. Once he was in the driver's seat, he made further changes. Since medicated women could not push their babies out, the doctor began to use

his forceps electively—to shorten the time of delivery—
which required the use of anesthesia. Coupled with this
came the practice of elective incision of the vaginal outlet (episiotomy), which also required the use of anesthesia. Thus, labor and delivery with the maximum
assistance of "modern science" involved sedation (twilight sleep) for labor, and, in most cases, anesthesia,
forceps and episiotomy for delivery. Childbirth had
indeed achieved the status of a surgical operation.

Of course it is true that abnormalities of childbirth
also came under close scrutiny, and solutions to many
of the problems appeared as medical practice advanced.
Anesthesia made possible safer surgery—the Caesarean
operation became safer—and the ultimate solution of obstructed labor was at hand. *All* babies could be born now
with relative safety to both mother and child. The
advent of blood transfusion brought with it a marked
decrease in maternal problems from hemorrhage. Greater
understanding of diabetes, Rh factor, and maternal heart
disease led to successful pregnancies for women for
whom it would not have been possible before. Great
investigations into the fertility and infertility of couples
were undertaken, and many formerly barren marriages
became fruitful.

The only victim of all these advances was the normal,
healthy girl with an uncomplicated pregnancy who just
wanted to have a baby!

For this girl, there came, in 1932, a lonely voice in
the wilderness. From England, Grantley Dick-Read began
to speak and write against many of these tendencies to
"improve" childbirth. He formulated an entire philosophy, upon which he then based a method of "natural"
delivery. "Childbirth is a physiological activity which is

closely associated with emotions. In the natural state the emotional experience of childbirth raises a woman to such delight and thankfulness that her mind turns to spiritual and metaphysical associations to satiate her expressions of great pride and joy. Whatever religion or gods are followed, it is seen and spoken of by those who believe and many who have never previously believed. . . . I am persuaded from long years of experience among women of many nationalities that good midwifery is the birth of a baby in a manner nearest to the natural law and design—and good midwifery, next to wise and healthy pregnancy, sets the pattern of the newborn infant and its relationship to its mother." [10]

Dick-Read embarked on his great adventure after a casual remark made to him after delivery by a poor woman in her home. When he asked why she had refused the offered chloroform—no one had refused him before—she replied that it had not hurt, and then added, *"It wasn't meant to, was it?"* And herein lies the basis of Dick-Read's philosophy. He felt that childbirth is a noble act, a beautiful emotional experience, and that such an act, terminating the miracle of reproduction, could not, in its divinely intended form, be profaned by pain.

Through the ages, he explained, fear and anxiety were introduced into pregnancy and childbirth. Fear and anticipation of pain arouse natural protective tensions in the body, both psychic and muscular. Unfortunately, the muscle tensions aroused tend to oppose dilatation of the birth canal during labor. This resistance causes pain by exciting nerve endings in the uterus that respond to excessive tension. Thus, fear begets tension, tension begets

[10] Dick-Read, G., *Childbirth Without Fear,* p. 12.

pain—a process that Dick-Read called the fear-tension-pain syndrome.

If this theory is accepted, then all one has to do is to overcome fear, eliminate anxiety and tension, and replace them with calmness and relaxation, and labor would be a wonderful experience. This is just what Dick-Read set about doing.

Since fear and ignorance usually go hand in hand, he instituted courses in "education for childbirth" so that the mother could understand and anticipate all that was happening and all that was yet to happen to her. The mysteries of labor and delivery were revealed, hospitals were visited beforehand, the professional vocabulary was explained. All of this was done in the hope of eliminating fear of the unknown from childbirth.

But this was only half of the job. A woman could approach labor with her fears controlled, with minimal anxiety about what was happening. But what about labor? How was she to deal with uterine contractions and expulsion of the infant? Wasn't this necessarily painful? Here, Dick-Read's theory dictated that relaxation was *most* important. The fear element must be reduced to a minimum, and tension must be thwarted during labor.

And so a series of "relaxation exercises" was devised. The objective was to achieve as complete relaxation— mental and physical—as possible during contractions, so that there would be no tension and therefore no pain. Proper breathing was important, since respiratory control played a large role in avoiding discomfort and helping the uterus carry out its work. (During the first stage of labor, respiration becomes deeper and more rapid as the intensity and duration of the contractions increase.)

Both abdominal (diaphragmatic) and upper thoracic (chest) breathing were taught. To help the expulsive efforts of the uterus, the woman was taught to hold her breath and increase her intra-abdominal pressure. After each expulsive contraction, she was taught to take two or three full, controlled, deep breaths, and to await the next contraction in a state of complete relaxation.

Thus the trained mother could go into labor understanding the phenomena that were occurring, trained in both respiratory and "concentration-relaxation" exercises to aid and supplement natural uterine forces. She was completely armed against the "fear-tension-pain syndrome." Why, however, go through all of this if she could receive an injection, sink into glorious oblivion and awaken a mother?

Dick-Read mentioned the benefits accruing to mother and infant from the least possible interference—of course, authors had written of this three centuries before. But for Dick-Read, there was another reason: Childbirth represented the acme of human spiritual achievement. ". . . the birth of a child is an emotional experience which brings with it all the noblest and most lovable qualities of men, women and children. It unearths the fund of tenderness, companionship and sympathetic understanding that smooths our social structure and brings confidence to replace suspicion. There is no greater joy than that of a woman who sees her baby born, hears its greeting and holds it in her hands while it is still linked to her body by the avenue through which its life blood surged from the selective source within her womb. The miracle by which new life is given to us has gained our highest respect, and we have seen, in awe, women pass from the physical to the spiritual comprehension of the magnitude of human love. . . . The care of the physical components of reproduction has for long constituted the main theme of obstetrics. But, no matter how carefully and apparently successful this may be, the raising of the standard of the human mind cannot be accomplished unless men and women are guided by the Creative and Directive Spirit." [11]

Dick-Read strongly resented the male attitudes of the medical profession, the imposition upon pregnant women of attitudes which discounted the aims and desires of the *females* who were pregnant. Needless to say, the writings of Dick-Read were widely read, and his ideas and methods were widely applied, with considerable success.

But, as with many other things, the gold of the method began to tarnish slightly as it was used over a long period of time. First, the extreme passivity required during labor did not suit many women. And then his techniques simply did not prepare women sufficiently well to cope with the physical discomfort of labor, since he denied the existence of discomfort. Finally, despite *his* ideas on the subject, it was difficult for many women to view labor as uplifting, beautiful, and spiritually rewarding.

Dick-Read's overwhelming emphasis on the great joys of childbirth was misleading. For many women, it just isn't so. It is impossible to measure the disappointment of those who did *not* have the subjective spiritual experience he describes.

There is no doubt that Dick-Read did much to open the eyes of the profession, to knock some of the veneer from the pompous, to liberate many women from what *men* thought childbirth was and should be. He showed that normal childbirth could be safely returned to the

[11] Dick-Read, *op. cit.*, p. 34.

mothers-to-be, who with some simple tools could manage quite well under supervision. And most of all, he removed the mysteries from childbirth and *restored the dignity of the laboring women*. Each woman in labor, as she enters the hospital, should murmur a soft thanks to Grantley Dick-Read; much of the way she has been treated and will be treated results from the writings of this great Englishman.

While the Western world was using, abusing, and refusing Dick-Read's method, it did not pass unnoticed in the Soviet Union. The Russians, however, made a different approach, a pragmatic approach that utilized Pavlovian psychology. Just as Dick-Read drew upon his background as a Westerner and as a Christian, so did the Russians draw upon their history, philosophy, and psychology.

In September of 1950 a World Congress of Gynecology was held in Paris. It was attended by delegations from many nations. Among the members of the Russian delegation was Professor A. P. Nicolaiev of Leningrad, who discussed a method of preparing women for labor that had attained huge success and popularity in the Soviet Union. Using principles of conditioned-reflex training, Soviet obstetricians and psychiatrists were preparing huge numbers of women for their labors and deliveries. These women were then able to deliver their children awake and with minimal discomfort. A French obstetrician, Dr. Fernand Lamaze, Director of Obstetrics for the Metal Workers' Polyclinic in Paris, was much impressed by what Professor Nicolaiev had to say, so much so that he joined a French delegation to the Soviet Union one year later.

On September 4, 1951, at the Institute of Obstetrics and Gynecology of the USSR Academy of Medical Sciences in Leningrad, Dr. Lamaze first witnessed a delivery conducted with psychoprophylactic techniques. He became so excited by the sight of a young woman actively working with her labor and relatively comfortable that he remained at her bedside for the entire six hours of her labor. During the rest of his first visit he watched the deliveries of more prepared women in both Moscow and Leningrad. He returned to Paris determined to implement this method there. This was done immediately upon his return, and within eight months most of the deliveries at the Metal Workers' Polyclinic were conducted using psychoprophylaxis. The success of the method quite naturally led to public controversy in France, controversy that frequently did not involve medicine and science so much as politics. But such controversy breeds publicity, and shortly women throughout France were becoming interested in the method of Lamaze.

Such was the dedication of Fernand Lamaze to the psychoprophylactic method that he personally carried the torch that spread the light through the Western world. By 1952 the technique was well established throughout the Communist nations, including China; Lamaze devoted himself to the enlightenment of the rest of the world. He first endeavored to adapt the "pure" Soviet techniques to Western custom, tradition, and standards of care. Further, he undertook the training of all obstetricians who came to him from whatever part of the globe. He thus provided a single center from which knowledge of and experience in the method could flow. Within the next several years, psychoprophylaxis became well established in more than forty nations of Europe and the Americas. The tremendous demand for the technique among Roman Catholic women raised theological questions. Pope Pius XII gave the method theological endorsement in a special audience for physicians in 1956, and a great hurdle was cleared. From then on it was clear sailing in Europe and South America.

But in the United States psychoprophylaxis had not made an impression. There was practically no publicity about the method and apparently little desire for information about it. "Natural childbirth" advocates used Dick-Read's principles and techniques, and there were several active centers teaching this to those who cared to learn. Dr. Isadore Bonstein of Geneva prepared women in Cleveland in psychoprophylaxis with good results, but that is as far as it went.

In 1959, however, the bomb finally burst over the United States. Mrs. Marjorie Karmel, an American woman who was delivered with psychoprophylaxis by Dr. Fernand Lamaze in Paris, put her experiences into a book, *Thank You, Dr. Lamaze*. Psychoprophylaxis had arrived in America. Within a short time, several obstetricians in the New York area began to use the method. When it became apparent that the method was gaining popularity, Mrs. Karmel conceived the idea of forming an organization devoted to the propagation of psychoprophylaxis throughout the United States. In conjunction with Mrs. Elizabeth Bing, one of the first teachers of the technique in America, interested obstetricians were contacted, and from their joint efforts the American Society for Psychoprophylaxis in Obstetrics (more commonly known today by its initials as ASPO) was founded in 1960.

Under the auspices of this organization—which now includes parents and teachers as well as obstetricians—classes in psychoprophylaxis have been set up in almost every major city, making available to mothers and the medical profession all possible assistance in psychoprophylactic training. It has been a long voyage since Dr. Lamaze met Professor Nicolaiev in 1950. But what has happened in those few years is all the more amazing for having occurred in so short a period of time.

VI

Principles of Psychoprophylaxis

What Professor A. P. Nicolaiev discussed in Paris in 1950 and what Dr. Lamaze witnessed in Moscow and Leningrad was a unique approach, developed by scientists and doctors in the Soviet Union, to the problem of pain in childbirth. Russian psychologists and psychiatrists had for many years been interested in hypnosis and its application to many of the problems in medicine, specifically to the control of pain. They became slowly disenchanted with hypnosis for two reasons. First, it was a technique that in many cases could be used only with great difficulty and with no reasonable assurance of success. Second, it did not get to the root of the pain or discomfort. What was the cause of pain; how was the response formulated? Hypnosis, when it worked, served only to supersede pain rather than to deal with the essential processes operating to produce it.

When, in 1930, Russian scientists were seeking a new approach to the phenomenon of childbirth, it was only natural for them to consider the theories of their contemporary Ivan Petrovich Pavlov, winner of the Nobel Prize and great physiologist. What Pavlov's work attempted was to discover the mechanisms by which people acquire information about the world inside and outside themselves and to explain what happens to this information and how the brain orders bodily responses appropriate to the information supplied. It was felt that a theory that could do this might easily provide a solution to the problem of pain in childbirth.

For many years before Pavlov and his group, reflex activity in man and animals had been studied by a wide variety of scientists. A reflex is an involuntary act brought about by the stimulation of a sensory nerve—for example, closing the eye when the lid is stroked is a reflex. Such a reflex act works as follows: A receptor—any specialized nervous tissue capable of receiving physical or chemical stimuli, such as eye, ear, touch receptors of skin, and pain and temperature receptors—is stimulated and transmits a signal via a sensory nerve to the brain, where the information is analyzed and interpreted and a response formulated. The signal for the response is then sent via a motor nerve to the appropriate muscles or glands for action. The signal from the brain can also be of nonaction, in which case the muscles do not contract, the glands do not secrete. Whether the effect is an action or a nonaction, the circuit, or "reflex arc," is the same: receptor, sensory nerve, brain, motor nerve, effector. Many investigators before Pavlov had explained human and animal behavior in theoretical terms using the reflex as the basis. However, the reflex had never been subjected to experiment in the laboratory. This experimentation was the contribution of Pavlov and his co-workers.

During the course of his research, Pavlov studied the salivary secretion of the dog. The production of saliva when food was placed directly in the dog's mouth was a reflex easily understood and explained physiologically. But Pavlov found that the mere sight or smell of food could evoke the same salivary and stomach secretion in the dog. This indirect stimulation of salivary flow—indirect because there was no direct contact between the signaling stimulus (odor or sight) and the responding organ (the digestive tract)—was not so readily explained. Having noted and described this phenomenon, Pavlov showed next that a dog that had been decorticated—that is, had had the highest, most well-developed, and most complex portion of its brain removed—would not react to the sight or smell of food, but would salivate only when food touched its lips. With the highest brain centers absent, the psychic salivary secretion was absent. Such a dog is deprived of its ability to survive, being unable to discover and distinguish food. It can eat only when food is placed in the mouth.

The next problem was to discover the origin of this type of response. Was the animal born with this pattern of response, or did it learn it after birth? The ability to salivate is inborn, but the signals in response to which salivation will occur are another matter. An experiment was constructed to answer this question. A group of puppies was isolated and raised on a diet of milk alone for more than six months. After this period the sight or smell of milk or milk products or the sound of splashing fluid evoked a salivary response; but neither meat nor bones nor other foods commonly associated with dogs could evoke this salivary response, except when placed directly in the mouth. The animals were indifferent to the sight, smell, or sounds of any food except milk. However, once other foods had been placed in the dog's mouth several times and were eaten, the sight, smell, and sound of these new foods also began to stimulate salivary secretion, a secretion indistinguishable from that formerly stimulated only with milk.

The significance of this experiment is great, for it demonstrates remarkably well that interpretation of the environment is *learned,* not innate. The animal learned through experience—exposure to certain substances as food—and then reacted according to its experience. The corollary to this most important observation was well demonstrated, too: Learned behavior can be unlearned, relearned, or modified in other ways by environmental changes.

The application of this experimental evidence to human behavior is quite simple. The analogy of food can easily be used. One need only look at the vast cultural differences in food to see that just as Pavlov's dogs were raised to eat milk and milk products only, so people establish for themselves food habits that are unique to their group and that they maintain and pass on. These patterns can become so ingrained that they are difficult to change even if survival is threatened. The experience of American troops in Korean prisoner-of-war camps is a good example. These troops were given minimal diets that included foods entirely alien to them, such as boiled fish heads. They were given little that could remotely be considered part of their previously experienced diets. The caloric intake provided by this diet was adequate for survival. What was needed was the ability to eat it! Most of those troops acquired this ability rapidly; some however, did not, and could not, therefore, survive. This ability to change or modify conditioned behavior is called adaptation.

Having shown that under normal conditions there are innate reflexes and learned (conditioned) reflexes, Pavlov now tried to evoke a salivary response in a dog by means of a stimulus completely unrelated to food—an indifferent stimulus. An experimental system was therefore devised in which the indifferent stimulus—the ringing of a bell—was applied at the same time as the administration of food. After several times, the sound of the bell alone became sufficient to evoke salivation. Neither food nor the odor or sight of it were necessary. Pavlov's famous dog, salivating to the sound of a bell, had been created. Pavlov called this reaction the "artificial" conditioned reflex.

The artificial conditioned reflex is part of everyday life in contemporary America. The entire advertising industry is devoted to evoking certain definite responses to indifferent stimuli. The brand name, an indifferent stimulus, is applied simultaneously with the product name in an attempt to replace the product name with the brand name and evoke the response of purchasing a particular brand. This has succeeded so well that certain brand names have almost become generic names—Frigidaire and Kleenex, for example.

Not only stimuli, but also responses can be artificial. Given a certain stimulus, different responses can be conditioned. Take the ringing of the bell, for example. The sleeping man turns off his alarm, the fireman reaches for his hat and coat, the sailor notes the time, the child salivates for ice cream—all responses artificially conditioned to the same stimulus. In discussions of artificial conditioned reflexes what is true for artificial conditioning of stimuli is equally true for artificial conditioning of responses. They are equivalent phenomena at opposite ends of the reflex arc.

There are, therefore, three different types of reflexes: the unconditioned reflex, the conditioned reflex, and the artificial conditioned reflex. The unconditioned reflex is inborn and unlearned—for example, salivation in response to the placement of food in the mouth, sucking by the newborn babe when anything is placed in its mouth. The conditioned reflex is learned or acquired—for example, salivation in response to the sight, smell, or sound associated with food, sucking by the newborn babe at the smell of milk. The artificial conditioned reflex is also learned or acquired but involves replacement of the "naturally" conditioned stimulus with an indifferent one—for example, salivation to the sound of a bell, sucking by the babe when picked up by the mother. It is on the theory of artificial conditioned reflexes that psychoprophylactic exercise techniques are based.

It should be apparent that both natural and artificial conditioned reflexes are based upon and derive from unconditioned reflexes. They are, however, not exact replicas of the unconditioned reflexes from which they derive. The stimulus in an unconditioned reflex is a broad complex of stimuli acting in concert in a given time that send powerful signals from a number of receptors to the brain. In the unconditioned salivary reflex, for example, the sensation of food in the mouth and its taste and smell all contribute to the signals sent to the brain. In the natural conditioned reflex, a smaller number of receptors respond to sensory impulses. Using the salivary example again, only sight and smell are available; the sensation of the food in the mouth and its

taste are absent. The stimulus complex is somewhat nar-
rower and, therefore, less intense. In the artificial conditioned reflex, the stimulus complex is reduced to a
single, indifferent stimulus—the bell, in the case of the
salivating dog. A single receptor, the dog's sense of hearing, now responds. Each of these stimuli evokes an identical salivary response, despite the marked difference in
stimulus complexity and strength. However, because of
this relative weakness of the stimulus in artificial conditioned reflexes, constant reconditioning of the artificial
pattern is necessary.

Pavlov described two broad functional areas of the
brain, the lower centers (subcortical) and higher centers
(cortical). Both centers perform useful and necessary
functions. The lower centers regulate the essential life
functions—self-defense, alimentation, elimination, sexual drives. Although it is necessary to maintain life, this
subcortical system never achieves a high degree of adaptation to the environment.

The higher centers consist of "analyzers" and connector paths to the subcortical centers, from which there are
connector paths to the various effectors. The analyzers
possess the two properties essential to the establishment
of a discriminating relationship with the environment—
analysis and synthesis. The organism selects, by analysis,
the significant stimuli from the totality of the environment, synthesizes a coherent stimulus complex, and
mediates an action according to this analysis and synthesis. The analyzers permit, therefore, the establishment
of a satisfactory relationship with the external environment. Through "temporary" connections (conditioned
reflexes), the function of the subcortical centers is modified, and a fine degree of adaptation can be achieved.

For example, if one is crossing the street without looking and suddenly sees a large bus bearing down, there occurs, without "thinking," a massive and immediate response of leaping back on the sidewalk, arms flailing. This is a true defensive reflex mediated through subcortical centers. It is appropriately wide and coarse, but unquestionably functional. However, should one step into the street and then notice the light change from green to red, one merely turns slowly and returns to the sidewalk. Here a fine adaptation to a small change in environmental conditions has occurred. The analyzer has detected the changed traffic signal as the important environmental stimulus of the moment. A synthesis then occurs, deriving the thesis that one should return to the sidewalk. Appropriate signals are then sent through to the effectors, and one slowly returns to the curb.

In order to permit an orderly and efficient analysis and synthesis, there are two important processes going on simultaneously in the cortical centers: excitation and inhibition, which are both actually sides of the same coin. Because all sensory receptors are constantly operative, many sensory signals arrive at the higher centers simultaneously. The stronger signals form stronger centers of excitation. These stronger centers of excitation inhibit the formation of excitation centers in response to weaker signals. Thus nonessential excitation is eliminated by this inhibitory mechanism—mental chaos is avoided and coordinated activity in one direction at a time is permitted. The importance during childbirth of this mental property and the necessity for functioning in only *one* direction at any given time will become evident later.

When he considered the higher, or cortical, centers of

man, Pavlov found that unlike animals, which can only respond to *real* stimuli from the immediate environment, human beings can respond to abstractions of reality through their unique faculty of speech and its comprehension. He therefore divided the higher centers into two parts, the first signaling system involved with the management of environmental stimuli from the receptors, and the second signaling system involved with "word" stimuli. Since words in and of themselves are not reality but rather abstractions from or representations of reality, Pavlov called them "signals of signals." Interestingly, however, words can evoke the same excitation of higher centers in human beings that real sensory stimuli do. Words, concepts, and ideas can thus enter reflex arcs and act as stimuli that are as powerful as any stimuli relayed from a receptor.

Pavlov's two systems are, of course, closely related, and transfers can be made of equivalent stimuli between them. Thus if a conditioned reflex to a real stimulus is established, the verbal representation of the stimulus can evoke the response as well. The opposite is also true: If a conditioned reflex is established to a verbal stimulus, the substitution of a real stimulus will also evoke the response.

An example of the transfer from a real to a verbal stimulus is the common response of anxiety to verbal suggestion that an injection is to be given. When some people are informed that they are "to have a shot," their pulse rate quickens, their palms become sweaty, they begin to breathe more rapidly and heavily. What has happened? Having previously had injections and found them to be unpleasant and perhaps painful, the conditioned reflex is established. A real stimulus, the prick of the hypodermic needle, evoked a bodily response—quickened pulse rate, sweaty palms, rapid breathing. Once this conditioned reflex pattern is established, the words "injection" and "shot," even when distant from the actual needle in time and place, evoke the same anxiety response. A word, concept, or idea has replaced the real sensory stimulus in the reflex arc. A "signal of a signal" has been formed—a conditioned reflex to a verbal stimulus has been established.

The theory of conditioned reflexes applies to childbirth in two ways. First, there are culturally conditioned stimuli—the attitudes, ideas, and concepts the mother-to-be brings with her to childbirth. Since these are verbal stimuli, they can be changed if they are wrong and truthful, forthright ideas can be substituted for them. Thus the attitude toward labor can be modified from great anxiety to calm equanimity. These modifications can be induced through intensive programs of prenatal education, in which, for example, one never speaks of "labor pains" but only of "uterine contractions." The entire conceptual milieu is calculated to establish as realistic and pleasant an attitude toward labor and delivery as possible. Thus when the real labor occurs it becomes part of a reflex arc carefully and thoughtfully prepared for it.

The second application of the theory is to the actual response to the uterine contractions of labor itself. There is no doubt that labor is associated with discomfort of differing degrees. When this phenomenon is subjected to analysis according to Pavlovian principles it can be thought of as follows: Receptors in the uterus are stimulated by uterine contractions. An impulse is sent to the brain via sensory nerves from the uterus. A center of excitation is then established in the appropriate analyzer and the impulse is interpreted as discomfort or pain. In accordance with the unpleasant interpretation, signals are then sent from the higher (cortical) centers through the lower (subcortical) centers to appropriate effectors, and the commonly observed mass response—writhing, moaning, and groaning—occurs.

Since this represents nothing more or less than a reflex arc, interference with and modification of this pattern are possible. In many reflex arcs, either the stimulus or the response can be subjected to conditioning. With labor, however, the stimulus—uterine contractions—cannot be modified; the uterus contracts involuntarily. There remain two ways to influence the reflex arc. First, it is possible to evolve an indifferent, conditioned response to the uterine contraction, a response mediated by higher centers and therefore finer and more delicate than the coarse lower-center response commonly seen. Second, the cortical mechanisms of excitation and inhibition can be utilized as well. If the cortical center of excitation required to mediate the conditioned response is made stronger than the cortical center of excitation aroused by the uterine contractions, inhibition of the uterine signal occurs. In fact, if the conditioned response occurs slightly before the uterine contraction actually takes place, it can prevent the very formation of the cortical center of excitation in response to the contraction.

A series of exercises has been devised to do exactly that. They are of increasing complexity—or, in Pavlovian terms, they require increasing intensity of cortical excitation for their performance. Being specific and directed toward the performance of highly integrated motor activity, there is no generalized subcortical inhibition, such as might affect labor. The subcortical motor responses are confined, and labor can progress unaffected.

These exercises, however, are just one part of the three-part approach of psychoprophylaxis. The other two parts are to decondition erroneous ideas about childbirth and to develop correct and worthwhile attitudes to replace them.

VII

———◆◆◆———

Erroneous Views
of Childbirth

The contemporary American woman is the victim of
her culture. It has beautifully conditioned her to a view
of childbirth that cannot serve her well when she enters
labor. Western culture generally, and American culture
specifically, considers childbirth synonymous with suffering. Uterine contractions are referred to constantly as
"labor pains." In movies and on television, women in
labor are depicted with contorted faces, sweating, grim-
acing, moaning, and groaning as though they were en-
during the very throes of hell.

All this makes it extremely difficult to approach childbirth with any degree of calmness or self-assurance. Yet
modern Western culture has perpetuated this attitude
despite its obvious uselessness and its frequent harmful-
ness. Why should this cultural phenomenon have occurred and been perpetuated? Furthermore, why should
this be such a mass phenomenon, common to such a large
part of the world? What began the insidious chain of
events that culminated in the widespread idea that

childbirth is suffering to be endured, not a normal bodily function to be performed?

Underlying any quest for an explanation must be the axiom that *normal, healthy* labor is *relatively comfortable* and *not too unpleasant;* that as a normal, healthy function of normal, healthy women, it should be undertaken with normal, healthy equanimity. Abnormal labor, on the other hand, is quite different. Here, a physiological and/or anatomical abnormality is present. The entire childbirth complex is functioning poorly. Such a situation is one of obstetric *disease.*

The reasons for this confusion of normal labor with abnormal labor are many. Probably the most important, however, is the information (or misinformation) transmitted directly from mother to daughter regarding the experiences of the mother in childbirth. "You must love and honor your mother, for I *suffered* to bring you into this world!" In days gone by, this statement must have had at least some basis in fact. Women then became pregnant at younger ages and continued to have babies through later years (there was no conception control) and under less favorable conditions. They were essentially unattended, only observed and comforted. Since little or nothing could be done to prevent or correct difficulties in labor, and since the conditions under which the labors were conducted were far from ideal, there must have been a fairly high percentage of abnormal labors. Unquestionably these abnormal labors resulted in pain and suffering for the women involved. This aspect of labor was readily observed and transmitted. Were not the normal, pleasant, easy labors, which represented the majority, also discussed? Probably not, because such things do not make good stories. If a woman says, "My, I had a pleasant and uneventful labor," she is apt to be answered, "So what?" Should a woman say, however, "Did I have a terrible time! They thought for a while I wouldn't make it!" the response would be "Really? Tell me more, what happened?"

The normal, healthy, usual, and therefore unexciting phenomena of life are not discussed; they are expected. It is the unpleasant, the unusual, the abnormal, the unhealthy, and, of course, the lurid that people discuss avidly. And, after much retelling, legend arises from fact. It is, of course, to these legends that young girls are exposed. They come from all sources: mothers, female relatives, movies, television, books. And the myth becomes the reality for millions of girls and young women who have yet to marry, become pregnant, and deliver a child—because the *words* can condition the reflexes necessary to make the myth reality. With this type of conditioning, what response to labor can reasonably be anticipated?

It might be expected that some social influences would tend to counteract these childbirth legends, would weaken their strength as conditioning stimuli. Alas, there are none. Instead, the prevalent stimuli relating to childbirth tend to reinforce these legends rather than contradict them. These reinforcing stimuli are essentially the male-dominated hospital obstetrics practiced in the United States. This approach dooms a woman before she starts.

A normal, healthy body function that must be conducted under the care of a physician seems, on the face of it, to be a contradiction. Furthermore, this normal, healthy function has to be undertaken in a hospital! These two facts are sufficient to reinforce the legends of suffering and agony in childbirth; after all, the ill and disabled who seek physicians' care in a hospital for relief of their malady are expected to experience suffering and agony. It would not be incorrect to say that prevailing opinion among obstetricians supports this contention, that they see themselves as rescuing unfortunate pregnant women from the "diseases" of their labors. They are further convinced that without their presence all would be lost, for they feel that they are necessary to labor and delivery in an active sense and that their interference in these processes is essential. So the obstetrician also reinforces the already prevalent view of childbirth as an unpleasant, abnormal evil, a disease. Who wants something like that?

To accept this view, however, is to mistake the frosting for the cake. Why go to an obstetrician when pregnant? Why deliver a baby in a hospital? Because though ninety-five percent of all pregnancies, labors, and deliveries are perfectly normal and would terminate relatively successfully for mother and child without assistance, five percent develop complications of one sort or another. Since one has no guarantee, at the onset of a pregnancy, of an uncomplicated course and termination, the purchase of "insurance" in the form of obstetrical care and guidance is prudent. And since some of the possible complications of labor and delivery may be catastrophic for mother and child, they can best be handled in a hospital. Thus to deliver a child in the hospital is also prudent.

It is therefore simply good sense to be under the care of an obstetrician and to deliver in a hospital. It is a realistic approach to childbirth that any reasonable woman should take. To deny the possible hazards of pregnancy, labor, and delivery, and to take a "do-it-yourself" approach, is foolhardy in the extreme. On the other hand, to surrender to the all-knowing doctor as does the person ill with pneumonia is unnecessary. The obstetrician should be considered merely an "insurance policy" against the small obstetrical risk.

Hospital routine and procedure are also guilty of reinforcing the idea that pregnancy is a disease. There are, as a rule, few differences in hospital processing of pregnant women in labor and hospital processing of sick people. Although maternity suites occupy their own floors, they are usually in the same buildings as facilities for the care of the sick. They frequently share admitting and administrative offices. It is unpleasant, to say the least, for a healthy, pregnant woman in labor to have to go to an office in which there sit sick people waiting for their beds. It is difficult for her to think she is healthy.

The pregnant woman in labor is also the victim of another aspect of hospital routine. A healthy person coming to a hospital for healthy purposes, she is completely deprived of visits by family and friends while in labor. The sick lie in coma surrounded by loved ones, while the healthy in labor lie alone. This confinement can be frightening. It has always appeared somewhat arbitrary to allow a husband to escort his wife to the labor suite, but no farther. Whether she had progressed to two centimeters of dilatation or ten at the time of admission mattered little. He could be with her only "on the outside." Fortunately this is slowly changing, and couples who have prepared for labor in formal courses of instruction may now remain united during labor and delivery in many hospitals. With this prospect in mind, the menace of the hospital atmosphere lessens.

Among the cultural influences conditioning women to

an unhealthy view of childbirth in the Western, Judaeo-Christian world is the Bible—the story of Eve. Biblical ideas of preordination, fate, destiny, seem to justify suffering in childbirth. Womankind is still paying for the original sin. Is this, however, a valid interpretation of the Bible? Is this really what religious thinkers believe today?

It was this very argument that was used against Sir James Y. Simpson when he introduced chloroform to England; it was considered immoral to alter God's plan. No official word was forthcoming from the Vatican until 1949, when Pope Pius XII sanctioned the use of hypnosis in childbirth. On January 8, 1956, speaking at an audience of European doctors on the subject of psychoprophylaxis, he said:

"A criticism of the new method from the theological point of view should in particular give an account of Holy Scripture, because materialistic propaganda claims to find a glaring contradiction between the truth of science and that of scripture.

"In Genesis (chapter 16), we read: *'In dolore paries filios'* ('In pain shall you bring forth children'). In order to understand this saying correctly, it is necessary to consider the condemnation passed by God in the whole of its context. In inflicting this punishment on our first parents and their descendants, God did not wish to forbid men to seek after and make use of all the riches of creation; to make progress step by step in culture; to make life in this world more bearable and better; to lighten the burden of work and fatigue, pain, sickness and death; in a word, to subdue the earth (Genesis, 1:28).

"Similarly, in punishing Eve, God did not wish to forbid—nor did He forbid—mothers to make use of means which render childbirth easier and less painful. One must not seek subterfuges for the words of Sacred Scripture. They remain true in the sense intended and expressed by the Creator, namely, *motherhood will give the mother much suffering to bear*. In what precise manner did God conceive this chastisement and how will He carry it out? Sacred Scripture does not say.

"It could be true that incorrect behavior, psychic or physical, on the part of those in labor is capable of increasing considerably the difficulties of delivery, and has in reality increased them.

"Science and technique, can, therefore, use the conclusions of experimental psychology, of physiology and of gynecology (as in the psychoprophylactic method) in order to eliminate the sources of error and painful conditioned reflexes, and to render childbirth as painless as possible. Sacred Scripture does not forbid it." [12]

For Roman Catholics, therefore, it is *not* the act of childbirth that constitutes the punishment of Eve, but rather the entire state of motherhood. It is *being* a mother that involves the pain and suffering, not *becoming* one. No longer need the Roman Catholic mother be bound by the myths of yesteryear. She has received papal sanction for her quest to make labor the rewarding experience it should be.

Contemporary Protestant theology and ethics view the Genesis story of Eve from two aspects. In the light of modern archaeological knowledge, the Bible can be looked upon as a work produced by unknown authors at a given point in history. Why was this story of the downfall of Eve and her subsequent punishment included?

[12] Pope Pius XII, "On Painless Childbirth," *The Catholic Mind*, pp. 288–89.

Dr. George Landes of the Union Theological Seminary in New York City feels that this may simply have been a way of explaining an observed phenomenon. Women apparently suffered in childbirth; here, then, was the explanation for this. If viewed in such terms, this story assumes the same significance as the mother-to-daughter transmission previously discussed, for it becomes merely a formalized attempt to *explain* this notion. Furthermore, this historical view of the story does not extract from it any concept of divine preordination or commandment that would doom women to inevitable suffering in childbirth.

There is, however, another side to the coin: The Old Testament has significance not only as literature, but as religious canon. The story of Eve represents the original sin and all that this connotes theologically. But, as Dr. Paul Lehmann of the Union Theological Seminary explained this for the author, the Genesis episode cannot be interpreted by the Christian as an isolated occurrence with an independent significance. For the Christian, the Old Testament can be interpreted only in terms of the New Testament. Thus, if Christ's death had, in fact, the significance ascribed to it, namely that He died for the sins of mankind, then through His death and resurrection, mankind achieved salvation.

Salvation means, according to Dr. Lehmann, that the "power of sin" has been broken through, so that now man lives by new and fulfilling possibilities and power. The story of Eve is a profound symbol of the depth and pervasiveness of sin and of the intimate connection—but *not identity*—between "original sin" and sexuality. Through the salvation brought to earth by Christ, this sin and its punishment no longer characterizes man's life and behavior in a fundamental and final way. In Christ, man lives under and by the reality and "power of grace," not under and by the reality and "power of sin." Thus the modern Christian woman is not destined to follow in the primeval path of Eve. No longer, therefore, does the main stream of Protestantism hold to the literal interpretation of the Bible. That view which enabled the clergymen of England to denounce Simpson and his chloroform as immoral is gone.

For the Jew, of course, the problem is completely different. Judaism does not have within its theology the concept of original sin. It regards national catastrophe and punishment as conditional on the deeds of man. "Behold, I place before you this day blessing and cursing. The blessing—if you heed the commandments of the Lord your God which I command you this day. And the cursing—if you do not heed the commandments of the Lord your God, and you turn away from the road which I command you this day, to go after other gods which you never knew . . ." (Deuteronomy XI, 26–28, translated by Rabbi Shulman.) Man must, therefore, do everything possible to make his life easier, while living the kind of life that will bring upon him God's blessing and not His curse. This concept governs personal life as well.

Therefore, the question of whether or not means and methods devoted to making childbirth a pleasant and pleasurable experience are moral does not even arise (as it obviously did for the Christian). For Judaic theology, there is only one proper course, and that is the prevention or the prompt and effective relief of pain and suffering by the most appropriate means available.

In fact, according to ancient Jewish tradition, the question of birth pangs is not even mentioned in the

Genesis passage. The words of the passage are literally interpreted by the Talmud to refer to "sorrow of raising children" and also the "period of pregnancy." "Your sorrow" refers to the process of raising children; "your pregnancy" refers to the hardship of pregnancy (Babylonian Talmud Erubin, 100b). It is evident that according to this interpretation the passage does not refer to physical pain but to mental anguish and to the normal parental hardships. Surely this is to be avoided whenever possible. The approach and aims of psychoprophylaxis fall well within this view.

Marxism, a "religion" lately arrived on the world scene, has a "theology," and one Soviet writer on obstetrical methods has attempted to reconcile the aims of psychoprophylaxis with Marxist ideology: "We must not forget that the beliefs, ideas and judgments of society are a superstructure on the economic basis. We therefore feel that we shall not sin against the truth if we assume that the man in the person of the chief of the clan, the slaveholder, serf owner, priest and minister of the cult also made use of painful labor for the purpose of securing and canonizing the 'eternal' difference between man and woman, the woman's 'uncleanness' and 'sinfulness' and 'lower position in society' in order to consolidate his right to exploit her.

"A good deal was also done in later times to fix in the mind of man the erroneous ideas that woman's inevitable suffering in childbirth was genetically conditioned and invariable." [13]

Thus, modern theology of whatever persuasion has turned against the myths of the centuries. Childbirth

[13] Velvovsky, I., *Painless Childbirth Through Psychoprophylaxis*, p. 165.

can now be viewed in its true perspective, and women are now free to seek means to make it the vital, meaningful life experience it should be for the mother.

And so the major conditioned attitudes toward childbirth in our society today have been revealed for what they are—perpetuations of mythology, misrepresentations of fact, and erroneous interpretations of Judaeo-Christian theology. With this knowledge, the strength of the conditioned attitudes wanes and healthy fact replaces unhealthy fancy. No longer need the narrow view and self-interest of some obstetricians obscure their real value and place. Childbirth can be safely returned to the mothers. No longer need Eve and her apple condemn a woman to suffering in childbirth. Childbirth is not divinely preordained to be painful.

Having considered some cultural errors of commission, it now becomes necessary to consider some cultural errors of omission. In its preparation of girls for womanhood, society has failed to prepare them for motherhood.

VIII

Educating for Childbirth

It is the paradox of our age that *pregnant* women must be educated in *pregnancy*. It is strange that there have been no provisions made to prepare young men and women for parenthood during the required years of formal schooling. The educational system prepares its products well for the demands and responsibilities of citizenship, for the scientific, intellectual, and commercial worlds. It prepares them somewhat for marriage and family life, but not at all for pregnancy, labor, and delivery, events that usually stem from marriage. To be sure, many high schools and colleges require a course in "hygiene" for girls, but what this generally consists of is some "between-us-girls" chatter on menstruation and occasionally a little about sex. Beyond some elementary discussions of mammalian reproduction with human applications, there is little or nothing made available to young women. For both men and women an important part of preparation for adult life is neglected.

Why should this be so in twentieth-century America? Why has such a situation been permitted to arise? First of all it must be realized that the need to provide more or less formal instruction in pregnancy is really rather recent: it is only with the increased urbanization of life, the limitation of family size, and the widespread acceptance and use of modern obstetrical care that the need has become acute.

When the American economy was primarily agricultural, people lived farther apart, in relatively isolated family units. The tie to the land and the necessity for human labor to work it made for large families. The mother became pregnant and remained at home in full view of all, cooking, cleaning, sewing, and so on. The young females of the household could see her and watch her pregnancy develop. They were necessarily aware of labor and delivery, for these phenomena would take place in the home with a doctor or midwife in attendance. They might also be called upon to assist in one way or another with mother or child. Thus young girls were quickly schooled in the "practical" biology of human reproduction, if not in its theory. Although their information was necessarily incomplete, their exposure was complete. They could not be told fanciful nonsense about storks and the like. As a result of their exposure to real pregnancy, their attitudes were realistic, and their fears, therefore, were realistic as well. It is obvious that one can control realistic fears based on valid information more easily than unrealistic fears based on ignorance. These women approached childbirth with greater calm and maturity, realizing the miracle that it is, rather than the mystery it has become.

Contrast this with modern-day urban life. Many individuals live isolated from their families in an urban sea of strangers. Though we live surrounded by people, we are biologically alone. As soon as possible one leaves the nest of home for boarding school or college or a job. One takes an apartment and lives in it alone. No longer are the young reared to maturity in the home, leaving only to establish a new family unit. They leave early and spend some of the formative years away.

Childbirth has also left the home and has gone to the hospital. What the youngster of today sees in the pregnant mother is a woman increasing in girth who visits a doctor periodically. She leaves one day and returns several days later with a baby and without a belly. Since all transpires away from home, there is no educational experience for the youngsters at home. They are effectively shielded from the labor and delivery, and nothing need be told them of the pregnancy except to prepare them for the new baby. So storks and similar prudish explanations become easy ways out for nervous parents.

Another aspect of rural life that contributed to greater understanding of reproduction was the presence of farm animals. Farm families bred and reared these animals, mated them, and assisted at the births. City folk have always felt that the attitudes toward sex of farm folk were rather "earthy." This was no doubt true once, for farm children observed and fostered animal sex—and the transition into human behavior was simple. Today, things are probably different for farm children too, for most animal breeding is now carried out with artificial insemination. Modern life has even upset the rural applecart!

The limitation of family size has also lessened opportunities for learning in the home about pregnancy, since there just are not as many people around from whom to learn. When families were large and all were at home, the older children learned from the parents and the younger children from the older ones. Today, with small families and separation from the home, there is no one to provide the example, to teach the lessons, to show the way. The child of today lives most of his waking hours in a world of his contemporaries—a world in which everyone is as ignorant and inexperienced as he is. Hence, the perpetuation of ignorance is to be expected. Where is this vicious circle to be broken, and by whom?

The resultant of these forces has been the aforementioned paradox—the necessity for educating *pregnant* women in *pregnancy* and preparing them for motherhood. But there is beginning to be heard throughout the land a clamor for knowledge. Women want to know and understand themselves; husbands want to know and understand their wives. There are those who would say that this type of education is nice, but is really a luxury. One injection and there is no labor and delivery. But it must be terrifying to approach motherhood with no knowledge of how to care for a baby. Through years of teaching classes for expectant mothers, it has become apparent that at least three-quarters of these women have never diapered, bathed, fed, or otherwise cared for an infant. If these women were left to their own devices, could they approach motherhood with peace of mind?

A woman desiring to prepare herself will find many excellent books available, filled with all she could desire (see the suggested reading list in this book). This is fine as far as it goes, but has the obvious disadvantage of being a depersonalized approach, and therefore it may not be adequate for some women. Also, the book cannot be asked questions.

Informal organized classes for expectant parents are to be preferred, for in such classes information can be provided by experts—doctors, nurses—who can be questioned and who can, therefore, tailor the material to fit the group. The most recent information and new trends and methods can be made available by such teachers sometimes years before they get into print. Also, the group setting provides other advantages to husband and wife. Since pregnancy is not a common condition among the population at large—the percentage of people that are pregnant at any given time is small—the pregnant woman in her usual milieu is most often the only pregnant woman. She is conspicuous and alone. Although she may be convinced that her state of being is normal, her differences are continually apparent. She may find it difficult to feel normal even though she knows intellectually that she is normal. Who feels as she does, has the same problems, fears, hopes, prayers?

Watch the face of a mother-to-be as she enters a class composed exclusively of pregnant women and their husbands. She relaxes, her face brightens. A communion has been achieved. Here she is not alone. Here she is inconspicuous. Her hopes, fears, prayers are the common hopes, fears, prayers. Her problems are the common problems. She can communicate, she can share. Now she is convinced not only in her mind but in her heart as well that she is normal. The creation of such a state of mind is important, for it sets the proper mood for the pregnancy.

Group training also encourages the participation of that neglected member of the team, the father-to-be.

Here is the fellow who will determine to a large extent the ease with which his wife will proceed through her pregnancy. His help, sympathy, and understanding are of incalculable value in sustaining the emotional health of his pregnant wife.

Most men feel self-conscious when they are made to become involved in a pregnancy. With his wife's going to a doctor and ultimately to the hospital, a contemporary male may decide his job ended when he contributed his germ plasm, and he may make believe nothing has changed until the baby comes home. There are, however, forces at work today tending to bring men back to their time-honored role as birth assistants, a role only recently abdicated. This unfortunate abdication has produced a generation of men whose ignorance of childbirth and its prenatal and postnatal aspects, exceeds even that of women. It is interesting to note that in meetings, classes, or other informal groups, the women are usually concerned with techniques and technical details, whereas the men seem preoccupied with "pain in childbirth." They sorely need the education offered in order to assume their proper role. When they are in the company of many men in the same situation, sharing the same hopes and fears, trials and tribulations, much, if not all, of their anxiety can be alleviated.

Group education makes the husbands more sophisticated helpmates to their wives. It makes it possible for wife and husband to experience the pregnancy and its events with mutual understanding, not just love. A husband cannot experience the pregnancy itself, but his ability to understand and evaluate events can assist his wife in her all too intimate involvement. Knowing that her husband can call her doctor, give an accurate description of uterine contractions or other phenomena, understand the answer, and do all this not with shame and embarrassment but with security and knowledge can be a source of great comfort to a pregnant woman. She is never really alone!

Psychoprophylactic technique calls for an attendant schooled in the method to be with the woman in labor and act as a sort of coach, timing contractions and keeping the woman doing the techniques properly. This coach (*monitrice* in French) provides a great deal of emotional support for the laboring woman. Ideally the coach should be the teacher responsible for training the woman, with the husband providing additional support. The shortage of trained teachers and the rules and regulations of some hospitals prevent the achievement of this ideal. The job therefore falls to the husband. Having attended the classes with his wife, learned the exercise techniques, and assisted her as taskmaster and critic in her preparation at home, he comes to the labor room well equipped to carry out this most important job when it counts most. Many a woman would have been unable to deliver her child awake, aware, and actively participating had it not been for the support, encouragement, and guidance of her husband.

Finally, there is a very simple reason for husbands to attend formal courses of instruction for expectant parents: Most metropolitan hospitals will not allow a husband to be with his wife during labor unless the couple has completed a recognized course of prenatal instruction. Some hospitals insist that the instruction be taken with them if the baby is to be delivered in their institution. Since not all of these offer training in psychoprophylaxis, it is occasionally necessary to take two courses!

Group training is directed toward the impending childbirth, preparation for labor and also parenthood. The biology of pregnancy, labor, and delivery is discussed in detail, and any and all questions that are answerable are answered. It is in these classroom sessions that conditioning begins. The word "pain" is discarded from the vocabulary. "Uterine contractions," the "sensation" of the "uterine contractions," and "discomfort" are the terms used, and the only terms permitted. The expression "labor pains" does not exist in psychoprophylactic preparation. By discarding the old emotionally charged and frankly disturbing terms, a whole new frame of reference is slowly but surely created. How much nicer when pregnant to anticipate a uterine contraction rather than a labor pain!

In addition, such matters as personal hygiene during pregnancy, heredity, breast feeding and care of the newborn infant are discussed. The groups are taken on tours of the maternity floor—labor and delivery rooms and newborn nurseries. This education (cultural conditioning and deconditioning) is coupled with training in physical psychoprophylactic techniques.

This type of preparation for childbirth and parenthood fills an educational vacuum. Labor loses its mysterious and frightening aspects while retaining its romance and excitement. The mystery of birth becomes the miracle of birth.

IX

Psychoprophylactic Exercises

Preparation and practice for childbirth should start eight weeks before delivery. If the training occurs much before then, some actual deconditioning occurs, and it is sometimes necessary to take a formal refresher session or two. One of the most important reasons for deconditioning is the loss of motivation. The longer from term one practices, the more easily the enthusiasm for daily practice wanes as the weeks drag on. It begins to seem as though labor will never occur. When this happens the maintenance of conditioning becomes more difficult. Therefore, should it be necessary to train early because of the scheduling of classes, plans should be made to take a refresher session or two with a subsequent group. Self-instruction and private instruction do not present this problem, of course.

How, it is always asked, can the psychoprophylactic responses be learned and practiced to a stimulus—labor—that is not occurring during the learning and practicing period? Furthermore, for mothers having their first baby, this stimulus has never occurred. Are they all, therefore, practicing in the dark, so to speak? The answer is, of course, not at all. All exercises are conducted and practiced by having an outside party (teacher or husband) say, "Contraction!" Then the exercise is performed and practiced in response to this verbal stimulus. It must be remembered that human beings have the ability to make ready transitions from verbal (abstract) stimuli to the actual stimuli they represent. Thus at the moment the first true uterine contraction of true labor begins, the transition of the stimulus from the word "contraction" to the actual physical sensation of the uterine contraction occurs. In Pavlovian terms, the first-order situation replaces that of the second order. If one has learned and practiced diligently, this transition occurs instantaneously and without difficulty.

The exercises that follow are divided into four actual training sessions. (Group training usually comprises six sessions, the first being an introductory session, the last a review.) Women learning at home should go through one session per week. Once the exercises have been mastered, practice should continue daily until labor begins. If this book is used in conjunction with an organized course of instruction in psychoprophylaxis, either privately or in a group, there may be slight differences between the organized course and the course described here.

Session I

Concentration Exercises

Before learning the exercises for the actual contractions of labor, the mother-to-be should learn exercises designed to teach control of specific muscle groups—to condition the ability to use specific muscle groups to the exclusion of all others. Although these exercises will *not* be used as such in labor, they are an important preparation for techniques that will be used. Repeat this series daily. The contraction and relaxation should be as complete as possible.

POSITION: Supine (on back) with a pillow under the head and one under the knees if desired; arms on floor slightly apart from the body.

EXERCISE:
Lift and contract right arm—relax
Lift and contract left arm—relax
Lift and contract right leg—relax
Lift and contract left leg—relax
Lift and contract right arm and right leg—relax
Lift and contract left arm and left leg—relax
Lift and contract right arm and left leg—relax
Lift and contract left arm and right leg—relax

Body-Building Exercises

These exercises will also not be used as such in labor. They are designed to help strengthen some of the muscle groups that will be used extensively in labor and also to help stretch the muscles of the outlet of the birth canal. This permits the baby to be born with less maternal difficulty. Each exercise should be repeated three to five times daily. In the performance of this series, always inhale through the nose and exhale through the mouth.

POSITION: Supine (on back) with a pillow under the head and one under the knees if desired; arms on floor slightly apart from the body.

EXERCISE:

1. While inhaling, slowly raise the right leg as close to the vertical position as possible. While exhaling, lower the right leg slowly to the floor. Repeat with left leg.

2. Place both arms on the floor, fully extended, at right angles to the body. While inhaling, raise the right leg as close to the vertical position as possible, with the knee straight. While exhaling, lower the leg slowly to the *side,* as close to the right hand as possible. While inhaling, raise the leg to the vertical position once more. While exhaling, lower the leg to its original position on the floor. Repeat with the left leg.

3. Bend the legs, placing the feet firmly on the floor. Press the small of the back against the floor, contracting the abdominal muscles at the same time. Hold for fifteen to twenty seconds, then relax.

POSITION: Seated upright on the floor.

EXERCISE:

1. While seated upright on the floor, place the soles of the feet together with the feet as close to the body as possible. Push the knees as close to the floor as possible with gentle manual pressure.

2. Sit cross-legged with the back slightly rounded, rather than straight. Assume this position as often as possible when pursuing daily activities.

Session II

Repeat concentration exercises.
Repeat body-building exercises.

Breathing for Early Labor

This breathing exercise is designed for use in early labor where the contractions are of low to moderate frequency (up to every five minutes or so), of short to moderate duration (thirty to forty-five seconds), and of low intensity. It should not be used merely because contractions have begun, but reserved for the time when control is actually needed. Since this is the simplest and *least fatiguing* of the exercises, it should be continued as long as possible—as long as it helps—before a more complex technique is employed. When practicing this and subsequent breathing exercises, the instructions "Contraction begins" and then "Contraction over" must be given by another person (husband) or you must mentally instruct yourself. The idea of contraction must be present in order to permit an orderly transition from the exercise as a practice technique to a means of controlling true labor.

Since there is a tendency toward drowsiness due to fatigue when in labor, all breathing exercises must be done with the eyes open and fixed on a simple convenient object in the room. Open eyes further reinforce the reality of the situation, thus helping to maintain the conditioned state.

POSITION: Seated comfortably in a chair, legs relaxed.

EXERCISE:

1. With the command "Contraction begins," inhale deeply, then exhale completely. (This is the so-called "cleansing breath" that should precede and follow each breathing exercise each time it is done.)

2. Begin slow, deliberate, rhythmic chest breathing, inhaling through the nose, exhaling through the mouth. Achieve a rhythm of six to nine breaths per minute.

3. When this is mastered, add rhythmic abdominal massage (effleurage) to the technique, performing it simultaneously with the breathing. With the onset of the contractions, the cupped hands, with fingertips resting on the skin, are placed at the lowest point on the abdomen (just above the pubic bone). While inhaling, stroke the abdomen toward the sides and upward to the level of the umbilicus. While exhaling, stroke downward in the middle. Thus a circular sort of massage is performed. This should be done simultaneously with the breathing, beginning with the command "Contraction begins" and ending with the command "Contraction over." To prevent irritation of the skin and hands, talcum powder

should be sprinkled liberally on the abdomen during the performance of this exercise.

If the sensation of the contraction is perceived primarily in the back, manual pressure against this area may be more helpful than abdominal massage. This can be done alone or by the husband. Occasionally, this sensation can be overcome by placing a bolster cushion (or rolled-up sheets) against the small of the back, grasping the head of the bed, and rhythmically, in time with the breathing, rolling over the bolster. The knees must be bent so that sufficient pressure can be exerted against the bolster.

Breathing for Well-Established Labor

This technique is next in order of complexity to the rhythmic chest breathing just learned. It should, therefore, be employed when the slow breathing has become ineffective. The technique will be learned in two stages, first rapid, shallow breathing of even rhythm (panting). Once this is mastered for periods of up to one minute, the actual method to be employed during labor can be practiced. Since uterine contractions occur in waves—that is, the intensity begins at a low level, rises to a peak, and then falls off—the rapid, shallow breathing should be done in the same fashion, accelerating with the contraction wave to the peak of intensity, then decelerating as the contraction subsides. When this is mastered, abdominal massage can also be added.

Occasionally some women become slightly dizzy when they first begin to practice this exercise. It is nothing to cause alarm. Tolerance develops rapidly, and the dizziness disappears. These exercises should be learned in both supine and sitting positions. Although most women prefer a modified supine position (with the back propped up) during labor, there are some who prefer to sit. Since one never knows in advance which will be the more comfortable, the techniques should be learned in both positions.

POSITION: Supine with two pillows behind the head and back and one pillow under the knees; or seated comfortably in a chair, legs relaxed.

EXERCISE:

1. On the command "Begin," take a deep, cleansing breath (inhale deeply through the nose, exhale fully through the mouth) and begin rapid, shallow, breathing (panting). Keep the breathing as superficial as possible, almost in the throat. There should, therefore, be little chest movement. On the command "Stop," take a cleansing breath and relax. This should be practiced until it can be done comfortably for more than one minute. Practice three times daily, twice each time.

2. On the command "Contraction begins," take a cleansing breath and begin slow, shallow breathing. With the command "Accelerate," increase the rate and maintain it at a rapid rate for twenty to thirty seconds. On the command "Decelerate," slow the rate of breathing gradually. On the command "Contraction over," take a deep cleansing breath and relax.

3. When this technique is mastered, add abdominal massage as previously described. It should be performed rhythmically, in time with the rate of breathing.

Session III

Review slow rhythmic breathing.
Review rapid superficial breathing.
Review accelerated and decelerated superficial breathing.

Breathing for Transitional First Stage of Labor

The transitional first stage of labor is the latter phase of the first stage of labor, when there are seven to ten centimeters of cervical dilatation. Here the contractions are at their peak of frequency, intensity, and duration. Women having their first babies have a more or less distinct transition only after which, with the cervix fully dilated, will they be able to exert voluntary expulsive efforts (pushing) with any effect. Since the baby's head is usually well descended in the birth canal, the pressure against the rectum is great and the desire to push occurs reflexively. This exercise is, therefore, designed to achieve two goals: it is complex enough and strong enough to overcome the cerebral excitation of transitional contractions and thus provides control of this stage of labor, and since it is impossible to push while doing this exercise, it thus overcomes the reflex desire to do so. For women having second or subsequent children, the exercise is necessary even for the short and poorly defined transition present. It aids, too, in controlling the desire to push when the tendency would be to push too hard too soon, causing the baby to be delivered too fast. When combined with proper pushing, and when both are properly used in response to the commands of the obstetrician, a slow, delicate and deliberate delivery can be achieved with a minimum of physical assistance.

POSITION: Supine with two pillows behind the head and back and one pillow under the knees; or seated comfortably in a chair, legs relaxed.

EXERCISE:

The technique consists of combining rapid, shallow breathing (panting) with regularly occurring forceful exhalations (blowing). The blowing is interrupted at regular, predetermined intervals, every four to eight superficial breaths. At the command "Contraction begins," take a cleansing breath; then begin rapid, panting breathing, four to eight breaths, then blow; four to eight breaths, then blow; four to eight breaths, then blow; etc. At the command "Contraction over," take a cleansing breath and relax. Practice three times daily for four or five contractions of sixty to ninety seconds each.

Session IV

Review slow rhythmic breathing.
Review rapid superficial breathing.
Review accelerated and decelerated superficial breathing.
Review "pant-blow" breathing.

Voluntary Expulsive Efforts (Pushing)

The uterus, through its contractions, is the only means of achieving cervical dilatation. Its contractions also cause a certain amount of descent of the infant through the birth canal. The uterine forces alone, however, are insufficient for the complete expulsion of the infant from the birth canal. They must be supplemented with the mother's voluntary expulsive efforts. As has been stated, the mother has an expulsive reflex because of pressure exerted on the rectum by the baby's head. However, the mere sensation of rectal pressure and the awareness of a desire to push do not mean that the optimum time and conditions for pushing have arrived. Push, therefore, only on command of the obstetrician. Through his internal examinations he will determine the best time to begin pushing.

The voluntary expulsive effort used to supplement the uterine contraction consists essentially of what is done in order to pass a constipated stool (bowel movement). The lungs are filled with air (this pushes the diaphragm down into the abdomen, increasing the pressure), the chest is tilted forward and the shoulders rounded slightly (forcing the diaphragm against the abdominal organs), while at the same time the abdominal muscles are powerfully contracted. All of these maneuvers serve to exert great downward pressure. The pressure would cause the passage of nothing, however, were it not for the simultaneous *relaxation* of the muscles around the anus. Thus one pushes, as it were, against an open door. In labor, however, there is a tendency to close the door, to tighten the muscles of the pelvic floor, constricting the vaginal outlet. This is essentially self-defeating, for it obviously retards the progress of the infant.

Training for expulsion, therefore, has two parts: learning sufficient control of the muscles of the pelvic floor to keep them relaxed at the proper time, and controlling and strengthening the abdominal muscles in order to exert proper and sufficient pressure.

Training Exercises for Expulsion

POSITION: Sitting in a chair, both feet on the floor, relaxed.

EXERCISE:

Contract the muscles of the pelvic floor as though *preventing* urination and defecation. (Do what you would do if you were urinating and wanted to stop in the middle.) Hold for several seconds, then relax. When standing or sitting, squeeze the buttocks forcefully together. Hold for several seconds, then relax. Practice five minutes at a time, three times daily.

POSITION: Supine with knees bent, feet flat on the floor.

EXERCISE:

Inhale and exhale normally through the nose. At the end of exhalation, forcibly blow out the remainder of the air in the lungs while contracting the abdominal muscles. Hold for several seconds, and relax. Take a cleansing breath. Do three times daily.

Training Exercise for Breath Holding

Since the contractions during which expulsive efforts will occur usually last longer than sixty seconds, training in breath holding is of some importance. Since no woman in labor can be reasonably expected to hold her breath for sixty seconds, it is best to accomplish the voluntary efforts in two or three breaths of twenty to thirty seconds each. The following exercise is designed for those who cannot hold their breath for more than ten or fifteen seconds. It will aid in training for longer periods of breath holding.

POSITION: Stand straight, heels together, arms hanging loosely at the sides.

EXERCISE:

Keeping the arms parallel, raise them forward and then upward to a position overhead, inhaling at the same time to the count of "one-two." Lower the arms slowly sideways to the original position, exhaling at the same time to the count of "three-four." Do twice daily for five minutes each time, performing the exhalation more slowly each time.

Method of Pushing for Delivery

POSITION: Lying on the floor with several pillows under the back.

EXERCISE:

1. As the contraction begins, inhale and exhale deeply through the nose. As the intensity mounts, inhale deeply and hold your breath. Place both hands behind corresponding knees, grasping the thighs firmly, while keeping the elbows well up and out to the side. Pull the knees up.

2. Place the chin on the chest, leaning well forward. Now contract the abdominal muscles forcefully and relax the pelvic floor.

3. Hold this as long as possible. When the need for another breath arises, move your head back, exhale, quickly inhale deeply, return to the former position, and resume pushing.

4. When the contraction is over, release the knees, lie back, take several deep breaths and relax.

5. If at any time your obstetrician instructs you *not* to push, use the "pant-blow" technique previously described.

6. Practice this once a day, but push for only a few seconds.

REMEMBER:

1. If possible, begin exercise training no more than eight weeks from your due date.

2. Practice diligently each day, following the plan outlined.

3. At least once a day, have your husband observe and criticize your performance of the techniques.

4. Have him give the commands so that he may become familiar with the procedure and so that wife and husband become a team. This is important for labor and delivery.

5. The techniques are simple; they are easy to learn and perform. But it is *hard work*. Your goal can be reached, therefore, only if you want it enough to work for it.

X

Awake and Aware

A few final comments are now in order to make certain that psychoprophylactic preparation for childbirth is understood for what it really is. First, it is obviously not "natural" childbirth. It is wholly artificial, a completely contrived and man-made way of dealing with uterine contractions in labor. The exercise techniques themselves should be coupled with the active support of husband, obstetrician and all others in attendance. The greater this support, the more successful the exercise techniques.

The psychoprophylactic method includes as well the judicious use of analgesic medications and techniques. By this is meant necessary use that aids in the relief of discomfort without impairment of consciousness, awareness, or ability to participate. If in the judgment of the obstetrician in attendance such medication is needed, it should be accepted. We have all attended women in labor whose tension, anxiety, and fear were so intense that the symptoms interfered significantly with the women's ability to perform the exercise techniques well. This led to inadequate relief of discomfort during contractions, which in turn led to more tension, anxiety, and loss of faith in the techniques. Judicious use of appropriate medication breaks this vicious circle and permits an orderly progression of labor to a successful and happy conclusion.

There still remain two important questions about the psychoprophylactic method. First, can it be used with induced labor? And second, is the method useful in cases of abnormal labor?

Since the exact hormone (oxytocin) that physiologically causes and maintains labor was discovered and preparations of it were made available, obstetricians have had at their disposal the means to initiate labor and maintain it through delivery. This is what is meant by having a baby "by appointment." When the time is deemed appropriate, the woman is sent to the hospital, not in labor. She is prepared, usually given an enema, and then small regulated amounts of oxytocin are administered, usually intravenously. Labor slowly begins and becomes well established. This labor, if studied in the laboratory by all modern methods of evaluation, is indistinguishable from labor that occurs spontaneously. This is not only objectively true, but subjectively true as well. It can, therefore, be readily managed by psychoprophylactic techniques. Psychoprophylaxis and induced labor can and do go together without impairing either technique. This means, of course, that should the administration of oxytocin be *necessary* in the judgment of the obstetrician because of some defect or difficulty with labor, psychoprophylaxis may still be the analgesic method of choice.

What about abnormal labor, the breech birth (where the baby is born with the buttocks first and the head last, rather than head first), the birth in which forceps have to be used? Can the exercise techniques still be employed? There is only one broad answer to these and similar questions. In any instance where it is feasible for the baby to be born through the birth canal, the exercises can be used with benefit. Furthermore, their help in preventing extraneous influences from affecting the subcortical centers mediating labor is even more important when an abnormality exists. Prepared mothers are cooperative, relaxed, and understanding mothers. Needless to say, this is of incalculable value when abnormality is present, perhaps of greater value than in normal births. With modern methods of anesthesia, in which injections of an agent can be given to numb the vagina and vaginal outlet, even forceps deliveries can be successfully accomplished in conjunction with psychoprophylaxis. It must be emphasized, however, that should any abnormality or possibility thereof exist, the judgment of the obstetrician should be followed without question. He is there to make such judgments. Trust him!

Psychoprophylaxis is *not* childbirth without pain! Although the approach can diminish the discomfort of labor and reduce it to manageable proportions, it cannot and does not eliminate all of the discomfort. To promise the complete elimination of pain in all cases would be false and misleading. Although pain is unpleasant and therefore usually undesirable, it is something all people experience at one time or another and can learn to bear if given the opportunity. Labor is unlike most pain in one respect: The contractions, and therefore the discomfort, are intermittent, not constant. The interval between contractions is always longer than the contractions themselves. One is, therefore, free of discomfort most of the time. If the discomfort can be diminished in intensity by psychoprophylactic techniques, the problem of dealing with labor is reduced to easily manageable proportions. It is common for women in labor to test the technique by allowing themselves one contraction without a breathing exercise. They usually never allow a second.

Psychoprophylaxis is a means to an end, not an end in itself. If learned well, practiced diligently, and applied properly, it can make available to any woman who so desires a childbirth in which she is awake, aware, and actively participating.

———•◆•———

The Mothers Speak

The only people who can attest to the effectiveness of psychoprophylactic preparation are those mothers who have used the techniques in childbirth. Who else can speak with true authority? For that purpose, the author has assembled reports by six different women. These mothers have various educational, cultural, and religious backgrounds. Three reports are of first labors, two of second labors, and one of a third. Although the reports speak for themselves, the author's comments have been included in italics to make these not only good stories, but illustrations of the practical problems of implementing the theory in practice.

Report 1—First Labor

On Christmas Eve 1962 at 11:18 P.M. I held a tiny newborn in my arms. I, the mother, had just brought a daughter, our first child, into the world. My husband

and I had realized a wish: to participate actively in the profound process that produced our lovely Katherine, to be present at her birth.

At a question-and-answer session following the showing of a movie on psychoprophylaxis in our class, a woman asked two questions: Why should I be awake for the birth of my child? How is psychoprophylaxis better than conventional procedures? My husband and I had answered these questions for ourselves. As human beings and artists (my husband is a dancer and musician; I am a singer) our approach to life is one of welcome. As people who have learned the nature of body discipline and all of its complex ramifications, psychoprophylaxis was appealing and logical. The conditioning value of practice was clear to us who know what an elusive thing is inspiration.

[*Despite the idealistic motivation of this couple, their approach is tempered with reality. They are aware at the onset that a great deal of hard work and diligent practice lies ahead. This awareness of the realities is all-important.*]

We practiced quite faithfully for about eight weeks before delivery. My husband and I developed a fine rapport, which stood us in good stead during labor. Hardest for me to master, and longest practiced, was the panting breathing. My tendency was to tense muscles in throat and shoulders as the pace of breathing increased, which threatened to limit my endurance.

I had an idea I was Mother Earth herself, that babies were destined to dance through my organs into the world. True, I'd had a buoyant pregnancy, had remained physically very active and felt strong. This image in mind, I was somewhat alarmed when amniotic fluid began to trickle—I was sure I'd be giving birth momentarily, on my living-room rug, perhaps. When I called my doctor in the wee hours, a groggy but nonchalant voice told me to "navigate as best I could" and to phone when contractions were spaced five minutes apart. The trickling of waters continued into the third day—the day of delivery. On that morning, contractions appeared with some frequency, but my husband and I were skeptical. It was hard for us to believe the day was at hand, impossible to realize that a thing so miraculous as a baby would soon appear!

[*Rupture of the membranes before the onset of labor occurs in normal pregnancies and need cause no alarm. The obstetrician should, however, be notified immediately and his instructions should be followed. Here it was deemed best by the obstetrician to do nothing and await the onset of labor. The couple was, however, reassured and could therefore wait the three days.*]

When I called the doctor that morning, he told us to be at his office at eleven A.M. and to bring my suitcase, "just in case." I didn't mention my qualms, mainly because I'd always made efforts to appear conspicuously levelheaded and hearty. I wanted to be "the type" for psychoprophylaxis. (Sometimes if you play a role long enough you become that character in reality!)

A cab ride uptown through Central Park was by turns tense and unreal, romantic and tender. Convinced I was entering the transition, I panted with each contraction. Actually, I'd encountered relatively few contractions at this point and was still getting to recognize them. Often I felt I'd missed the onset of the contraction, jumped on the train while it was leaving the station. I raced through a cleansing breath, raced after a contraction which itself was speeding to a peak of intensity. My husband, calm and sure, carefully reminded me to breathe deeply after each contraction. We linked arms, incredulous at what seemed to be happening.

At the doctor's office we learned how far labor had progressed: The cervix was effaced (as indeed it had been for several weeks), still thick, and dilated a mere three centimeters. He urged me to return to shallow thoracic breathing, to hold panting in reserve as long as possible. Since I knew where I was, I reinterpreted the sensations and returned to shallow breathing easily.

[*This is a common occurrence with first labors—believing that the labor is further along than it really is. The contractions are misinterpreted in the newness and excitement of the moment. The only problem arising from this is that the woman tends to use, too early, unnecessarily fatiguing techniques—panting, in this case—when simpler and less tiring techniques would suffice.*]

My husband, my doctor, and I spent a charming hour chattering like old friends at a tea party. Each contraction resulted in a new spurt of amniotic fluid. I continued to breathe and rub my belly with the contractions, which were entirely bearable, partly because of their terminal nature, and largely because I could do something active while they lasted.

[*Even in this early part of labor, the fact that she was armed with something to do during contractions was all-important.*]

At one P.M. my husband and I had lunch: I was permitted clear soup. We'd been instructed to meet the doctor at the hospital at four P.M. and to distract ourselves meanwhile at the Metropolitan Museum of Art. Armed with a large box of sanitary napkins to catch the

fluid, we walked—more properly, I lumbered and wad-
dled; I was "great with child"—to the museum.

[*It was deemed advisable by the obstetrician for this
couple to stay away from the hospital during this early
first stage of labor. They were, however, in touch with
him, and were therefore not unobserved.*]

Greek vases, Oriental rugs, Degas bronzes—we saw
them all through eyes informed by our unique situation.
They all seemed symbols of fertility and creativity. At
length I switched again to panting. The fluid, not to be
contained, began to trickle down my legs. I didn't feel
like walking, contractions seemed more intense, I'd lost
interest in ancient artifacts. Again, I feared giving birth
momentarily—under a pot or behind a statue. I was self-
conscious about the panting and belly massage. In spite
of my discomfort, my spirits were high. I felt as if I were
being whirled to the center of things, into the "heart
of darkness."

At three P.M. we headed up to the hospital. Contractions were now coming every three minutes, lasting a
minute and sometimes a minute and a half. At half-past
three we met our doctor and the next phase of the adventure began.

[*This mother was admitted to the hospital at this
point because by now her labor had become well established.*]

In the labor room I was "prepped" by nurses, who
were completely cooperative. [*"Prepped" is hospital jar-
gon for shaving the pubic hair.*] As soon as they saw me
breathing *à la* psychoprophylaxis they understood I was
a "natural" case and suspended their work during contractions. The only real ordeal, and perhaps the most
trying of my labor, was the enema. Bodily sensations of

all varieties were visited upon me in great overlapping waves! I was sure the jig was up—I couldn't feel a contraction until it was at its peak. But no—as soon as the enema had done its work, I returned to mine, although I trembled for a while.

[*The "ordeal" of the enema is one of those unfortunate necessities. There is no way to make it comfortable; it must merely be endured. It is given because an empty lower bowel means that no fecal matter will be expressed from the rectum as the baby is born.*

With the knowledge that she has an empty bowel a mother is not afraid to push when instructed, for she knows that she cannot "move her bowels," which might embarrass her. It is important to note again that the mother can easily reinterpret the sensation of the contractions when she knows where she stands in labor.]

Now my husband and the doctor arrived, both clad in green sterile gowns. These two were my constant companions, my supporters, each a *sine qua non!* We joked, we talked, they encouraged me, reassured me. More than anything else, I needed this companionship—my husband, calm, loving, concerned; and the doctor, jovial, beautifully casual ("You're only having a baby!") and informative. Both were very, very kind.

The cervix was dilated to four centimeters at five P.M., and at the urging of my doctor I returned again to shallow breathing, again reinterpreting the sensations. It was, by this time, quite easy to detect the onset of contractions (the baby thumped a bit as forewarning). I sat in a chair through most of seven hours spent in the labor room. This position suited me better, psychologically, than reclining, and I preferred a brightly lit room. [*Comfortable positions in labor vary greatly from woman to woman. Prepared mothers are usually permitted to do as suits them best.*] With each contraction the conversation about me faded in proportion to my concentration, like a radio turned down. I withdrew into my task, fixed my gaze on a glass bottle nearby, rubbed a tummy covered by the soft muslin hospital gown. I found it helpful to sway rhythmically, too, and rotate my head loosely about on its axis. These movements seemed to relax muscles in the torso. While I didn't have back labor, my husband rubbed my back—the whole back—because it feels wonderful. [*She added a few frills of her own to the standard exercises, and to good advantage!*]

Around six P.M. an internal examination revealed the cervix to be dilated five centimeters. Panting at this point seemed to suit the contractions better. It was easier to breathe in this manner than it had ever been during practice, and I felt I could continue indefinitely. Now I sucked a lollipop.

[*Her progress in labor is quite normal for a first labor.*]

At nine P.M. the cervix still remained at five centimeters. A few membranes remaining in front of the baby's head were ruptured. I was fatigued and somewhat discouraged. When a nurse remarked, "Doctor, your psychoprophylaxis patients always do so beautifully in labor," I greatly appreciated her words. Yet I found it difficult to relax between contractions, tensed my body during them, and felt generally irritable. There was a slightly irregular presentation of the baby's head, which made me think labor would be endless and the expulsion greatly complicated. My doctor offered to administer a small dosage of Demerol and gave me time to think it over. He assured me its effects would be to hasten the progress of labor and to relax me. Thoughts of failure, of lost control, of intensified labor—all of these plagued me. Yet I took the Demerol, fifty milligrams in two doses of twenty-five milligrams each. He stressed that I was "still the same woman," words I'll not easily forget.

[*This mother had been in labor for more than ten hours by this time. The excitement and fatigue combined to make her a bit tense. For that reason a small dose of Demerol was administered to break the cycle caused by tension. She required reassurance, however, that she had not failed by having Demerol.*]

Demerol turned the trick. In two and a half hours the cervix was completely dilated, during which time I responded almost robot-fashion to contractions and relaxed well between them.

[*With relaxation from the medication, her labor once again proceeded well and quite rapidly.*]

Toward the last, contractions were spaced two and a half minutes apart and lasted from forty to sixty seconds each. Interestingly, at no time during labor could I respond intelligently to the question, Have you noted a change in the character of the contractions? I was able to observe more easily changes in my responses to the contractions—an increasingly vigorous effort was required to control them. Possibly, since work output must equal the intensity of each contraction, a sense of change is neutralized.

At nine centimeters of dilatation we became very excited. If I had been drowsy, I was now wide-awake and ready for the final effort. I felt great pressure as the baby entered the birth canal, and I responded, under the guidance of my doctor, to the urge to bear down. Panting and blowing out nicely controlled the urge when it was desirable. With each push my husband and the doctor were able to see a little more of someone's curly head. So there really was a baby to be had out of this!

[*The small amount of medication helped! It did not impair consciousness or the ability to participate in her childbirth.*]

I bore down with exceeding vigor—even broke blood vessels in my face. In fifteen minutes, at eleven P.M., I was ready for delivery. All things I had been led to expect regarding delivery-room procedure now occurred, and with astounding rapidity. [*Nothing in the delivery room was strange to her.*] My doctor appeared gowned in delivery-room blue. Leggings and other clothes were placed over and on me, with a small opening remaining through which the baby would emerge—"like viewing the birth through a window"; the phrase came to me from somewhere.

I continued to bear down on command, pant-blow on command. These moments were supercharged; I was working at peak concentration. I could feel and visualize the little body sliding up to the vulva, feel the tremendous stretching of the perineum. My style of pushing changed somewhat: I arched my back and threw my head back, bore down on the diaphragm using leverage afforded by the hand grips. My breathing was very loud, and I felt compelled to announce that, truly, I was not in pain, just terribly out of breath.

[*In order to avoid an episiotomy (incision of the vaginal opening) she was instructed by the obstetrician how much to push, when to push, and when not to push. She states that she was not in pain. This is characteristic of second-stage contractions.*]

When the birth of the head was literally "at hand," my doctor cautioned me not to fear tearing, that it wouldn't happen. In truth, I did indeed feel my very foundations giving way—the earth was being torn asunder, hell was harrowed. But I welcomed, with a most primitive pleasure, this immense catharsis. Labor's hurling and whirling had planted me starkly over against the inevitable.

[*The immense stretching of the skin about the vaginal opening gives the sensation that it is about to tear apart. Forewarning and reassurance usually solve this little problem.*]

The three of us, the doctor, baby, and I, performed a neat *pas de trois!* The doctor gave commands, I obeyed. With each push the perineum was stretched just a bit more until the baby's head was eased through with only a small mucosal tear, which was quickly sutured. Nineteen pushes in thirty-eight minutes.

My courage to look at the newborn head failed me! I waited until half of the torso had emerged. The child was incredible to behold—beautiful in every way, folded like a new butterfly, crying heartily even as her little legs slipped into the world. My husband had witnessed it all, happily standing in the doorway of the delivery room, and was greatly moved. I had a further surprise when my doctor gave me the wet infant to hold while her umbilical cord was cut. Then came the placenta, with a few more pushes.

[*The placenta usually separates with three or four postdelivery contractions, which are hardly perceptible, and can be easily expelled by the mother.*]

Later, in the delivery room, too excited to sleep, I turned the day's journey over and over in my mind, reliving, as indeed I do almost every day now, the moments of labor and birth. There were misgivings: Had I elected to be present at a ritual too sacred, too intense to assimilate? Had I trespassed upon territory reserved for the detached professionals and for the gods themselves? I wondered how my *spirit* would survive the extreme stretching and expansion it had undergone.

Across the hall another woman was laboring alone, totally anesthetized. Her cries were heartbreaking. The dignity, beauty, and rightness of my child's birth suddenly became clear. I had been the key participant in an enormous rite, the rite of passage. I am changed: My eyes have seen, my heart has known, I am now a woman in a new and fuller sense—a mother.

Through psychoprophylaxis, these great moments were made possible. I don't really consider my experience to have been "painless," yet the contractions were at all times entirely endurable because I was able to do something about them, to cope with them in very specific ways. [*Note that it was not "painless," but quite tolerable nevertheless.*] I agree heartily with those women who have noted that labor is hard work. In some ways it is the hardest work I have ever performed! I was extremely fortunate to have been under the care of a doctor of great skill and sensitivity. He helped us to use psychoprophylaxis in a way that best suited us, our physical and emotional needs. Any method should be flexible to accommodate the individual cases to which it is applied; psychoprophylaxis, it seems, incorporates flexibility.

Finally, I look forward eagerly to the birth of my next child, whose coming into the world will surely be equally, if not more, inspiring. I am moved to proselytize, to spread the word among my childbearing friends.

Report 2—First Labor

At my weekly visit to the doctor at 3:30 P.M., Monday, he examined me and said that the baby's head was partially engaged and the cervix was about eighty-five percent effaced and slightly dilated. As my due date was still a few weeks off, I wondered if all this meant that I might deliver sooner than I expected. My doctor told me that it was quite possible that I would stay as I was for a few weeks or that I could deliver soon. [*This was not a hedge by the obstetrician, but merely a statement of fact. It is not possible to predict with accuracy at this point.*] I reported to the doctor that I had been having rather frequent irregular contractions since that morning. I had had these contractions all during the latter part of my pregnancy, and except for the increased frequency they were no different from the previous contractions.

After leaving the doctor's office, I went downtown to do some shopping. I returned home at 7:30 P.M., and aside from being tired I felt fine. I was still having contractions, but it wasn't until 11:15 P.M. that I felt a vague cramplike discomfort with one of the contractions. My husband had come in from school, and I told him of the visit to the doctor and mentioned that I was feeling a little bit different than usual. We went to bed and at 1:30 A.M. I awoke from a deep sleep, aware of a terrible backache. As I gathered my senses I also became aware of the contractions, which came about every ten minutes and were like mild menstrual cramps. The contractions lasted thirty to forty seconds. I remained in bed and was fairly comfortable as long as I kept my fists under the small of my back. Although I did not sleep I was able to relax and rest until early morning. [*She is now noting the onset of true labor, which awakened her. The contractions have become regular with radiation of the sensation to the small of the back. Having been prepared, she was not alarmed. Thus she spent several hours relatively comfortably.*] Around five A.M. the contractions became more frequent and seemed to last longer. I put on the light, picked up my watch and the book I was reading, all set for the ritual of timing the contractions. My husband woke up, and when I told him that I was in labor he said, "Really?" and promptly went back to sleep. [*This is a common response of prepared husbands!*] The contractions were occurring every four to five minutes and lasted forty to fifty seconds. I was still comfortable and did not start the exercises. At 5:15 I had a blood-tinged mucous discharge, and whatever doubt I still had as to whether or not this was it vanished. I went back to bed and read until six, when I called the doctor. I told him just what was going on and he said that we could meet him at the hospital at 7:30. [*Her preparation enabled her to make an accurate estimate of her status and give an accurate report to the obstetrician.*]

I fully agree that it is unnecessary to awaken your husband if you start labor in the middle of the night, but I now think the husbands shouldn't be told this. At 6:30 I told my husband that if he was to get dressed and have a quick bite to eat he ought to get up; he very lovingly replied that it was so nice in bed, why didn't I get back into it!

We arrived at the hospital, met the doctor, and went up to the labor room. After the examination the doctor told me that I was five centimeters dilated. The contractions were coming about every three to four minutes, lasting fifty to sixty seconds and becoming more intense, although I still did not begin the exercises. [*This mother is now in well-established labor, having progressed to five centimeters of dilatation, but still felt no need to begin exercise techniques.*] After I was admitted, my blood pressure, pulse and temperature were taken by the nurse. I was shaved and given an enema. I went to the bathroom to expel the enema, and this was the only time I thought that I would never survive. All at once I had a contraction, started vomiting (fortunately I had remembered not to eat), and was expelling the enema. [*Again the "ordeal of the enema." Her vomiting is not unusual. Nausea with or without vomiting is a frequent occurrence in the first stage of labor. For this reason women are instructed not to eat if they feel that they are going into labor. It is also advisable to have an empty stomach should the necessity arise for an anesthetic.*] After about fifteen minutes I was able to get into bed and my husband came into the room. At this time I began to use slow breathing and effleurage (abdominal massage). The doctor examined me about 9:30 and told me I was six centimeters dilated. The contractions increased in intensity and duration to sixty to seventy seconds, still occurring every three to four minutes. About 9:45 I switched to accelerated-decelerated breathing without really thinking about it. [*Notice her orderly progression from slow breathing to accelerated-decelerated breathing as the contractions become more intense.*] From this point on it became vital that my husband loudly call out the passing seconds during the contraction and that he apply pressure to the base of my back with his fist. Without his help I would not have been able to maintain control. At 10:15 the doctor ruptured the membranes, a procedure that caused me no discomfort. The contractions became very intense, lasting up to ninety seconds every three minutes. I was eight centimeters dilated, and when the doctor asked me if I wanted to push I said no. With the next contraction, however, I suddenly had the overwhelming desire to push. I sent my husband dashing for the doctor, who was just outside the door. He examined me and then uttered those magical words: "You can push now."

[*A very clear example here of the onset of the second stage of labor. As the cervix dilated fully she felt the sudden urge to push.*]

I found it very uncomfortable to push with the bed elevated but didn't think to ask anyone to lower it. [*In the excitement of the moment many women forget to have the bed adjusted.*] The doctor had told me that I would feel like I was going to come apart but to do as he said. After four contractions with pushing I was taken to the delivery room on a stretcher. My husband was able to see the baby's head but then had to leave, as he was not permitted in the delivery room. It was 11:30. I was put on the table, my feet were placed in stirrups, and I was draped. I had three contractions in the delivery room and was able to do as told except with the contraction with which the baby's head was delivered. I was a little slow to stop pushing, as I was panting instead of blowing and there is a vast difference between the two results. [*She had some difficulty in controlling the urge to push because she failed to use the recom-*

mended pant-blow technique. In this instance, however, it made no difference.] In a matter of seconds I saw the baby being born and observed that it was quite obviously a little girl. She was a real deep bluish purple, a little cheesy and screaming, but beautiful. [*Babies are normally this color at birth, changing to their characteristic pink after they have taken several breaths.*]

She was born at 11:38 A.M., and the placenta was expelled shortly thereafter without any discomfort or difficulty. At 12:15 I saw my husband as I was on the way to the recovery room. He had already seen the baby, and one of his first comments was that her nails needed to be trimmed.

In conclusion I would like to jot down a few scattered thoughts. I was a little surprised by the sudden increase in the intensity of the contractions following the enema and the rupture of the membranes. The backrub and the timing of the contractions were essential, as was having ice chips to suck. I vomited once during transition, but at that point I think all self-consciousness and modesty went to the winds, because I was too busy to notice where the sheet was or who was who. [*This describes common reactions during labor. Many women report this.*] I also lost all sense of time, and everything seemed to be happening so fast that I was getting confused. The only remark I made to the nurse who took me to the recovery room was that I would gladly do it again that afternoon, and I meant it. I am eagerly looking forward to another baby and another happy experience with psychoprophylaxis.

I did not have an episiotomy and took no medication. [*A first baby delivered without an episiotomy! Possible but not common!*]

Report 3—First Labor

Being an expectant mother for the first time, I was naturally curious about what childbirth would really be like. After hearing about psychoprophylaxis, I found it exciting to believe that I could actually participate and see the birth of my child. I think there are many women who would like to participate in this joyful event but who are fearful because they have heard so much about the aspect of pain in labor. I must admit I myself had this concept before I attended the prenatal program. This course included the psychoprophylactic method. In this course we learned to concentrate on breathing techniques during our contractions. My husband and I were educated about childbirth in these classes. We also became aware of what we could actually expect to happen and what to do during the various phases of labor. The more we attended these classes, the more relaxed and sure of ourselves we both became. [*The effect of conditioning!*]

Then came the much-awaited big day. I could hardly wait to see what the much-discussed *contractions* would actually feel like. Finally I awoke one morning with what felt like mild menstrual cramps, which came invariably every eight minutes. After timing these contractions for about four hours, we telephoned the doctor. He asked if I could meet him for an examination. I was examined and told to come back in about four hours (which would be about eight P.M.) for another examination. I was also told not to eat any solid foods. [*The examination revealed only early labor not requiring hos-*

pital observation. As before, solid food was withheld to be on the safe side.] During this time the cramps were still at the same eight-minute intervals and had the same intensity. I remembered from the lectures in class and from readings that I should not start my breathing exercises until it was absolutely necessary to do so. Since I felt no real need for them, I refrained from doing them. After my examination at eight P.M. I was told that actual labor was not far off. I was advised to return home until contractions were no more than five minutes apart. Contractions were now beginning to feel a little sharper.

[*She was sent home again because reexamination revealed progress insufficient to warrant hospitalization. This prolonged period of contractions with little progress in cervical dilatation is not uncommon in first labors. It is usually called prodromal labor. It was also experienced by the mother in the first report.*]

My husband and I returned home to watch television. By this time I was beginning to feel tired. I dozed off for a short nap until approximately one A.M. About this time contractions were beginning to feel like something other than menstrual cramps. They were becoming more intense and lasting much longer. They were now four to five minutes apart. We called the doctor to report this change and were told to leave for the hospital.

After arriving at the hospital at about two A.M., I found it necessary to begin breathing techniques. I began with the slow-breathing exercise preceded and followed by a deep inhalation-exhalation. I was taken to the labor room and prepped, then joined by my husband and the doctor. At this time I was trying to make myself as comfortable as possible. I found sitting in the chair very relaxing.

[*With progression of the contractions in frequency
and intensity, true labor had unquestionably begun.
Breathing techniques now became necessary. Here is another mother more comfortable in a chair. There is
nothing sacred about laboring in a bed!*]

It was now about five or six, and the doctor had returned to break the bag of water. About this time I had
advanced to a more rapid breathing technique. I was advised that delivery would not be too far off. I now found
it more comfortable lying down, as the contractions had
increased in frequency. My husband began rubbing my
back, which gave me quite a bit of relief in that area.
He reminded me that maybe a change of breathing
would also be more relieving at this time. I now began
the pant-blow breathing although I had no urge whatso-
ever to push.

[*After the obstetrician artificially ruptured the membranes (broke the bag of water) to enhance labor, she
was more comfortable in bed. Her husband did his job
as coach very well by suggesting a change of technique.*]

It was now about seven A.M., and by this time I could
hardly believe I was actually going through with what
I had been practicing for almost two months. The
breathing techniques were actually working. Before and
after each contraction I was busy concentrating on the
cleansing breath. Without the help of my doctor and
husband, I often wonder if I would have been so successful. [*The importance of teamwork by mother, husband,
and obstetrician cannot be overstated.*] They were both
wonderful and very encouraging. They gave me the feeling that it just wasn't a job for one person, but that we
all had certain parts to play.

At eight A.M. I had begun perspiring quite a bit. My

mouth had now become so dry that I was given ice to chew. I was now waiting for the phase of labor where you have the urge to push. I cannot remember having so much of an urge. I was feeling sleepy by this time and found myself sleeping through contractions. [*No medication was given to this mother, but she had slept very little the night before and naturally felt sleepy.*] My husband was standing over me reminding me of my breathing techniques. My doctor had been examining me off and on all through the night and reporting to me how many centimeters I had dilated. It was now time to push the baby through. I could not believe that this moment had finally arrived, but I was asked to begin pushing when the next contraction began. I started out with the cleansing breath when the contraction started, then I held my breath to push. This was very exciting to me, because I was now able to push the baby far enough so the head could be seen. I did this a few times and before I knew it I was ready for the delivery room. Everything happened so fast after entering the delivery room that I can hardly remember everything. [*This mother also vividly describes the excitement of the second stage and the apparent rapidity with which it passes.*] I was asked to push again about two times, and the next thing I knew the doctor was holding up my baby. I was so busy watching the cleaning of the baby that before I knew it the afterbirth was ready to be expelled. I gave one push and it was all over.

I was given the baby to hold. This must be one of the most wonderful moments a woman could ever experience. All I could do was to admire this child with thankfulness—thankfulness for many things, one of them being that I had helped bring my baby into the world.

Now, months later, I am still talking about psycho-prophylaxis. I am so happy with the success of this technique that I feel I could never accept any other form of childbirth unless it was absolutely necessary for me to do so.

[*This is an unquestionably successful outcome. She was pleased with the delivery and would like her other babies to be delivered the same way.*]

Report 4—Second Labor

After a normal pregnancy, my husband and I were impatiently looking forward to the delivery of our second child. It has always been one of my strongest convictions that the final experience of pregnancy should be shared and enjoyed by both husband and wife. And now this dream would be almost fully realized.

After the birth of our first daughter I had heard about psychoprophylaxis, and I became quite interested in one day using it. My husband began to share my interest and finally became very enthusiastic at the prospect of working together at this time when our anticipation was the greatest. I believe that the easy and uncomplicated delivery of our first child and my continuing enthusiasm for childbirth influenced a change in my husband's feelings.

[*The experiences related by this mother are not unique. Many women have an initial problem of interesting a husband, but once the men are interested, their enthusiasm may exceed that of their wives.*]

Although I had not been trained in psychoprophylaxis with our first child, I had wanted my husband with me for reassurance. However, our daughter was born in a military hospital, and since military babies are almost mass-produced, there is no room for sentiment. Husbands don't belong. At this time, my husband was relieved. He was still thinking in terms of "suffering," and he couldn't bear to see me suffer. I couldn't convince him that I had no intention of suffering and I couldn't convince the military that my husband belonged with me. And so our daughter was born amidst strangers. I must say here that although the delivery was quick and without complications, it was a very lonely experience.

[*Her first delivery took place "amidst strangers" and she felt lonely—a situation the psychoprophylactic method seeks to avoid. She had had excellent, modern, scientifically correct care; but this* science *had failed to give her a* human *experience.*]

And so, although this was our second child, we were looking forward to it with as much excitement as the first, since my husband would now have an active role. Our course stressed that it would be necessary for husband and wife to understand their roles and practice working together so that at the time of delivery, reactions would be automatic. I can't say that I didn't worry a little bit—I worried about practicing enough, I worried about whether it would work for me, I worried about panicking, I worried about embarrassing my husband.

[*These worries, so well described, are not uncommon— they are the logical things about which to worry.*]

We decided that I should have induced labor. Of course, I worried. Finally the day of delivery arrived and I summoned my courage (not for delivery but for the intravenous injection used for inducing labor), and off to the hospital we went. I felt like a student at college again—cramming for that one exam I should have studied for and didn't. I practiced those exercises over and over for fear that I would forget them.

[*Induced labor was decided upon because this mother had to arrange for someone to look after her first child before she and her husband could both be away from home. Again a problem of modern America, where people live far from family and deliver their babies in hospitals. Only if all is prearranged can a mother have a second child with her mind at ease. Induced labor has proven to be a blessing to these mothers.*]

After the necessary preliminaries my doctor arrived and the process started at 9:50 A.M. I must have pestered my doctor with a million questions. How soon does labor start this way? I'm hungry! When do I eat? Will you have a lunch tray ready for me? Should I feel strong contractions? And so on.

I would like to say that I had a very easy labor. I did the deep-breathing exercises for a little while, but could completely eliminate them if I was engaged in conversation. Often while I was diligently doing my deep breathing, my husband and my doctor would begin discussing something amusing. Believe me, it's impossible to deep-breathe and laugh at the same time. I laughed.

[*There are apparently stimuli other than breathing exercises that can cause strong centers of cerebral excitation.*]

At last came the panting. At home this was the source of my greatest concern. I didn't seem to be able to do it for any length of time. Would I be able to do it when I had to? My husband had more faith in me than I had

in myself. I can't begin to express how important it is
to learn to work with each other. Whenever I tensed,
one word from him was all I needed to relax. [*This
mother, as well, emphasizes the need for close teamwork
among the three members of the team. At this point the
husband was foremost, later the obstetrician. She needed
both, however, each at his time.*] Previous concern completely left me at this point, and the panting seemed to
come easily. Unlike the deep breathing, panting could
not be eliminated. However, I only used this twice when
I began to feel the urge to push. Upon examination, my
doctor found that I had dilated about eight centimeters
and decided that I would be more comfortable in the
delivery room.

[*With second labor it is possible and frequently desirable to begin pushing before the cervix is completely
dilated. In these labors, pushing can assist in the com-
pletion of dilatation as well as in expulsion.*]

This was the final lap, and so far everything had progressed easily and normally. Unfortunately, husbands
were not allowed in the delivery room, so from here
on I had to depend on my doctor's reassuring words
and instructions. Once in the delivery room, I was allowed to push whenever I felt the urge unless otherwise instructed. At that point I would have to blow as
hard as I could until I was allowed to push again. This
was a little more like the work we were told about in the
course. I think I might have become a little panicky
had it not been for the calming words of my doctor.
I can recall that the urge to push was so strong at one
point that I was afraid that it might overwhelm me.
However, with his words of encouragement, my doctor
managed to reassure me, and consequently I was able to

keep as composed as the situation would allow. At
11:58 A.M. this very hungry mother was seven pounds
and fourteen ounces lighter and ready for lunch.

It was wonderful being with people who knew of the
method and approved. It made things much simpler. I
felt that it had to be successful for me, not only because I
wanted to see the birth of our child, but also because
I couldn't let these people down.

[*It is important to notice the strong effect the positive
supporting attitude of the staff had on this mother.
However, her expressed attitude is precisely that against
which psychoprophylactic education and training is directed. The motivation should come from within, not
without. Childbirth is not and should not be a performance to gratify any audience.*]

It was so very different from when our first child was
born. There was no anesthesia this time, so there were
no aftereffects. To be conscious and to see our baby's
birth was a feeling that I will never forget and never be
able to explain. It's a glow and yet it's more.

The entire experience left me with a deep feeling of
satisfaction and a desire to continue having children in
this relaxed and yet dignified manner.

Report 5—Third Labor

Both of my first two deliveries had been under complete sedation, although before the birth of the second
child I had heard of psychoprophylaxis and had brought
Mrs. Karmel's book, *Thank You, Dr. Lamaze,* to my
doctors' attention. They expressed doubts about certain
aspects of it and generally discouraged my interest. Un-

fortunately, I did not seek out a doctor who was more sympathetic.

[*The experience of being discouraged by doctors un-sympathetic to this approach to childbirth is all too com-mon.*]

I had no anesthetic for this third delivery, nor did I have any nausea, vomiting or grogginess, all of which I'd experienced in varying degrees with the first two.

[*Since this was her third baby, certain specific benefits of psychoprophylactic delivery appealed to this mother. She had sufficient experience for comparison.*] My husband was amazed that this time, twenty minutes after giving birth, I could pull myself up on my elbow to look at the baby with him and then reel off names and phone numbers of people he should call. It was quite a contrast to the scene after the birth of our second child, when he'd arrived two hours later to find me barely coming out of the anesthetic, groggy and hilariously incoherent.

[*The lack of aftereffect of anesthesia is all-important to the mother. Remember there is a lack of aftereffects for the baby as well!*] This time I felt tired and a little shaky for perhaps half an hour in the recovery room, but by the time I got to my own room, I was ready to sit up, brush my hair and think about dinner.

After the earlier deliveries, I had taken several days to get back to walking and sitting comfortably. This time, however, I experienced no soreness in the leg and thigh muscles and absolutely no discomfort in moving or sitting. I am sure that this was due largely to the exercises taught in the class I attended, although the lack of an episiotomy also contributed. It is certainly signifi-cant that I felt no need to take the "pain pill" offered at bedtime the first night. The only slight stiffness I had was in the arm muscles, caused by pulling hard on the hand grips during the expulsion. The vulva and perineum felt as though they had been stretched, but this caused no discomfort, even in sitting, and disappeared within a couple of days.

The labor did not deserve the name for the first two and a half hours (half its total length). After that—by then the membranes had been ruptured—the contractions began to strengthen, although their length and the intervals between them remained nearly constant until delivery. [*Notice once more the change in character of the contractions after rupture of the membranes. This change must always be anticipated.*] I began the slow breathing, the effleurage, and finally the panting, as each seemed necessary. The panting is much easier than when done in practice sessions. It becomes a reflex, and as the contraction strengthens, one automatically increases the rate of breathing.

[*Her experience that panting is easier in actual childbirth than in practice sessions is certainly the usual one among trained mothers. Difficulty is anticipated, but rarely materializes once the contractions of true labor begin.*]

The transition was difficult. By this time, I seemed to feel the contraction almost entirely in the groin and as back labor, exerting very little force in the upper abdomen. I can remember being glad to get each contraction over with and dreading the advent of the next, and I am sure that this led to a build-up of tension. I wish I had expressed these feelings at the time; perhaps then my doctor or my husband could have helped me to relax more completely.

[*One cannot emphasize too strongly the necessity and*

desirability of making the true state of comfort known to
the obstetrician. Without this information nothing can
be done.]

Things happened too fast once we got into the delivery room. The peculiar position on the table was much more comfortable than I'd expected, but I was hit by a sort of lightheaded feeling, accompanied by a terrific outbreak of sweat. Somebody wiped my face off, and about this time I was told I could start to push. I never did have any identifiable urge to push. [*It is not unusual to have no great urge to push at this stage of a third delivery. Thus the delivery itself and the ease with which the doctor's instructions can be followed are facilitated.*] Certainly I pushed, and hard, during the expulsion contractions, and it was very satisfying. But I had no great feeling of wanting to start to push and did not have to restrain myself from pushing at the wrong times. I think it took only about four expulsive contractions for the head to be born, and I was able to follow my doctor's instructions to lie back and pant, which I had expected would be very difficult to do.

As the baby was born, the two resident doctors who were in the room helped me to sit up more than my propped position allowed so that I could see the actual birth. I am not the kind of person who gets ecstatic about things, but I did feel very happy (perhaps I'd have been ecstatic if it had been a boy—this was our third girl), and I can remember grinning, it seemed, from ear to ear as I lay back and watched what was going on in the room around me.

This was not a painless delivery. Just a few minutes before the baby was born one of the residents had asked me about the pain. I put him off, wouldn't admit that there was any, although I was under stress and certainly uncomfortable at that particular moment. But that was labor—hard work, something to be done. The pain was brief, probably just at the crowning and the birth of the head. Perhaps if I had been able to be more relaxed there would have been none; I know women who have had psychoprophylactic deliveries and maintain that they felt nothing to describe as pain. [*This section should be read and reread, for it describes in words only a mother could write the essence of the experience. It was not painless, but she went through it with little difficulty and it turned out to be interesting and rewarding. One could not ask for more or receive more!*]

I found the whole experience interesting and rewarding. It is so much better to know exactly what is going on, and to feel that you have some control over it, than to have to let things happen to you. My husband and I both found the classes we attended informative, and I was glad to have reaffirmed some of my own ideas about maintaining normal activities during pregnancy. The exercises taught were very helpful, I am convinced, in preparing for delivery, and also I found them refreshing during pregnancy, on days when I was tired and could not manage time for a nap. The delivery was more difficult than I had expected, but I would certainly do it again this way. I am only sorry that I did not have my first two children with psychoprophylaxis.

Report 6—Second Labor

A report on this birth begins for me with a brief account of my experiences when my first baby was born in England in November 1961. I had trained myself in the psychoprophylactic method with the aid of a record and books. The baby was to be born at home, and I had explained what I was learning to my doctor and midwife, who were quite sympathetic. Unfortunately, both were away on the night when my labor began and I was left temporarily in the care of a pupil midwife. This girl made a mistake in determining full dilatation, and having used the Lamaze techniques extremely successfully up to this point, I was made to push on an incompletely dilated cervix for nearly three hours. This of course resulted in an obstetrical emergency, and I was taken to the hospital not understanding at all what had gone wrong—and I was criticized by the doctor on duty for not having been sedated at the beginning of labor and told that this had delayed the birth and endangered the baby's life! I could not continue the Lamaze breathing and relaxation techniques in this situation. I abandoned them and rapidly got out of control through pain and fear. I was sedated sufficiently to deprive me of all self-control but not enough to give me any relief from pain, and for two and a half hours I fought and screamed during a forceps delivery that I still remember in vivid detail. I was dominated by a terror of losing my baby and feelings of guilt at my early request not to be sedated. Because of my mental condition afterward I was given a truthful explanation of what had really hap-

pened. I was very deeply affected indeed by this childbirth, and it was many months before I regained my
self-confidence. I used to wake in the night screaming
for many weeks afterward. (I should not like this dis-
aster to be considered in any way typical of English midwifery, which is generally, I think, of a very high standard.) [*This account of an exceptionally bad experience
with a first labor and delivery is important, because this
mother brought very unfortunate memories with her to
her second labor.*]

This experience did not make us lose faith in the psychoprophylactic method, because the early part of my
labor had proved its value. I felt, however, that I could
not face another birth without a doctor who understood
the method. I was anxious to be able to have a baby
while living in New York, because such a doctor would
be more easily found there than in the remote north of
England. I was reasonably confident during my pregnancy and enjoyed the training classes, although I was
disturbed by being reminded of the impending birth
and had to fight off memories of my first confinement
after every class. In particular it was an ordeal to practice
the exercises for the expulsive stage of labor. However,
my husband and I worked very hard at the breathing
and relaxation exercises until I was again proficient at
them. [*The memories of 1961 were with her throughout
her training and even affected her ability to practice. She
went on, however.*]

My due date was March 3, but it was found when I
was examined on February 18 that I was already dilated
three centimeters. An appointment was made for me to
be admitted to the hospital on February 22 for induction
of labor. However, in the early hours of February 19

I was awakened by contractions that were irregular but strong enough for me to do regular slow breathing while they lasted. They continued at irregular intervals (twelve minutes, fifteen minutes) until I noticed a blood-stained discharge at 8:30 A.M. My husband had already left for Manhattan, and as I was very anxious to get within reach of husband, doctor and hospital as quickly as possible, I drove myself to the school from our home. We called our doctor and then went to the hospital. By that time, the contractions were less frequent, but I was found to be dilated four centimeters, and an oxytocin drip was used to induce labor at 11:15 A.M. [*This mother was in early labor, but since the contractions were relatively ineffectual for the degree of discomfort they presented, labor was stimulated with oxytocin.*] Regular contractions began immediately and were of forty to sixty seconds' duration at three-minute intervals. By doing the slow breathing I was only aware of them as a tightening in the abdomen. I had difficulty in detecting the beginning of the contraction at first, as my uterus felt hard to me at all times. My doctor assisted me by showing me where to place my hand to feel the hardening of the muscle. Soon after these contractions were established the membranes were ruptured artificially during a contraction. (This was at 11:45.) This procedure seemed to me painful and unpleasant, and I was quite unable to relax while it was being done. I found every examination during a contraction difficult, because in addition to the inevitable discomfort one is exposed to some extent to the pain of the contraction itself.

[*This is a common problem during labor. Both the examinations and the contractions can be unpleasant. Is it better to combine them and thus get it all over with at once? Many obstetricians prefer to examine during a contraction, since more information can be obtained and fewer examinations are necessary.*]

I was prepared for stronger contractions after the membranes had been ruptured and had no difficulty in adjusting to them. (I had been somewhat apprehensive about having an induced labor, as I had imagined that it might proceed at a speed difficult to control. However, this was not a problem. The only difficulty came in inserting the drip into my arm, as my veins proved to be somewhat elusive and the drip had to be removed and replaced several times. Once in position, it was comfortable and did not restrict my arm movements.) I now began to use rapid superficial breathing during the contractions, which at first lasted for fifty seconds at two-minute intervals, then for sixty seconds at two-minute intervals. [*Notice how she changes her breathing techniques to conform to the contractions.*] There was some irregularity in the rhythm; for a while they lasted for seventy-five seconds at intervals of two and a half minutes. At this stage I felt the contractions as a much stronger squeezing in the abdomen with no painful sensation. The ceiling of the labor room was white with black indentations that looked like geographical features and provided a useful point of focus. I had no difficulty at all in keeping up the rapid breathing and very slightly modified the rhythm I had practiced at home. It had been suggested at the classes that we should synchronize the effleurage and panting by allowing eight pants for the hand to travel from the pubis to the navel. I did this and also slightly emphasized every eighth pant, at the point where the hands were about to begin a new downward or upward movement. I found this of great benefit in keeping a steady breathing rhythm both in practice and in labor.

I was extremely dependent on my husband throughout the first stage of labor for his help in timing the contractions and especially for giving me five seconds' warning before one was due to start. I felt this dependence very much when my husband and doctor left me a little after one P.M. to have a sandwich and coffee outside the room. Although I was only alone about ten minutes and could hear their voices all the time, I found it much harder to synchronize breathing and concentration without help. During this period I became confused and mistimed one contraction, which was painful. There was a clock on the wall, but I could not concentrate on it. [*The importance of the husband cannot be overemphasized. Notice what a difference his ten-minute absence meant.*]

After my husband came back the contractions grew considerably stronger, and when I passed about seven-centimeters of dilatation, they began to acquire a painful sensation, as though my groin were being gripped in a vice. This caused me to tense my legs during contractions. I also had a backache. I continued to experience these difficulties until the end of the first stage of labor. I changed to the breathing for the transitional stage and also asked my husband to count off every ten seconds until the peak of the contraction had passed. At this point the contractions came every two minutes and lasted only fifty seconds. The peak was over after forty seconds. I think now that I could have done more to lessen the discomfort during this phase. [*This mother too states that more might have been done to enhance her comfort if only she had mentioned it.*] I had become rather hypnotized by the mountains and canyons on the ceiling, which had probably outlived their usefulness to me. Also I was stuck by habit, perspiration and amniotic fluid in the thirty-five-degree position I had assumed, and I was accepting as inevitable the tension in my legs instead of trying to do something about it. I discovered very belatedly that I was much more comfortable leaning forward with knees bent outward and eyes focused in a downward direction.

I think I made the mistake at this point of being too passive. To combat this tendency when actually in labor to forget some of the advice one was given in training, it might be a good idea for the husband to take a few written notes with him to the hospital, which could be checked from time to time. I think too that I was so absorbed in keeping on with the breathing that I did not give much indication to anyone that I was having difficulty at all. Several nurses were observing my breathing at this point, and this was an added incentive to maintain a relaxed air, because I was anxious to give a good impression of the method.

Nevertheless, the pain I felt was perfectly bearable, and at no time did I feel my control threatened. I did not once groan or become generally tense. At about 1:50 P.M., when I was dilated eight or nine centimeters, I was moved to the delivery room. It was then that I discovered I was more comfortable in a sitting position. [*Many women find it more comfortable to labor sitting in a chair with their feet on a low stool.*] I was shown every consideration during the move and allowed to stop and breathe when necessary. I think that this was important; a failure to time contractions properly when they are very strong could be very unpleasant.

[*Moving in between contractions is important. If faced with nursing personnel who do not understand this and try to move you while you are having a contraction, refuse to move. They will learn quickly enough.*] After being placed in position on the delivery table I was asked to push on the next contraction to hasten full dilatation. This was an unexpected development and made me feel apprehensive. It was rather painful to push, and I became tense at the further examination required. I was suddenly reminded of the sensation of pushing on the undilated cervix in my first confinement. I began to lose confidence and became very reluctant to push. However, after only three or four contractions the cervix was fully dilated and I began to feel the pressure of the baby's head. This also recalled my previous delivery, and I remained very tense. I was terrified of losing my self-control. [*The entire state of anxiety felt by this mother in the delivery room is understandable in the light of her previous experience. But all forces joined to subdue this noxious influence and to help her carry on.*] Despite this I held my breath and pushed during the contraction, though I felt that I was not being very effective. I was unable to relax between the contractions and forgot to keep my eyes open and take cleansing breaths. I was very surprised when I was told that the baby's head could be seen, and once again my mind reverted to my previous delivery, when I had been lied to on this point. Of course I believed the doctor this time, but I could not get rid of my preoccupation with my memories. At the height of my anxiety another patient began screaming in an adjoining room, and this helped me. I felt intensely sorry for the woman and realized that I was not suffering at all by comparison. After that I pushed with a little more courage, though I remained tense to the end. I was fortunate in having my husband present in the delivery room, and he helped me to lift myself up to push. While the baby's head was being delivered I found it a relief to stop pushing and return to panting and blowing. I did not find the delivery of the head especially difficult. I experienced greater discomfort a minute later from the sensation produced by the still-unborn body. At the moment of birth I was anxious about the baby's well-being and was afraid to look in the mirror. [*Her underlying tension throughout this phase of labor is understandable, but she rose above it.*] However, he cried as soon as his head was born and was soon placed on me, crying very vigorously. My husband and I were so happy to be able to watch his first moments of life together!

On analyzing the experience afterward I knew that I had not felt any pain as such during the expulsive contractions. Instead I had had to make a great physical effort accompanied by some discomfort and much anxiety and tension. I did not have any sedation or anesthesia at all during my labor—it would have been irrelevant to my difficulties. [*Notice how she feels that sedation or anesthesia would not have solved her problems.*]

It seems to me to be very important to overcome the handicap of a traumatic delivery when training for a subsequent birth. In dilatation the woman has time to prove to herself that the method is going to be effective as she successfully controls the contractions. During the delivery there is no opportunity to experiment. The physical and emotional sensations are so tremendous that if one is not completely controlled there is a danger of feeling engulfed. [*This analysis is of great value. Read it carefully.*] In dilatation the techniques appear to work the same way for all properly trained women (apart from the back-labor problem), whereas one's approach to delivery is probably determined much more by individual temperament and experiences, one's ideas about birth, and hopes and fears for the baby. It may therefore require a very intensive effort to decondition a patient from unfavorable attitudes to delivery.

Immediately after the birth I was disappointed that I had become so tense during the delivery, but on later reflection I knew that the birth had been a deeply rewarding experience. I felt well, sat up and talked and ate a meal soon after the delivery. I had chosen ward accommodation, and some of the other patients were Spanish-speaking. I suspected that I was something of a puzzle to them, since one, a Cuban woman, came over and asked if I had had a baby! [*This mother's comparison of her experience and resultant attitudes with those of untrained women deserves to be read and reread.*] I had not been in the room half an hour before I had guessed the Spanish for "pain" and knew that they were discussing their bad experiences. There followed five days in the atmosphere of traditional childbirth—the newly delivered mothers being brought in, prostrate and silent for hours, as I had been after my first confinement; the endless recitals of painful ordeals and the affirmations of "never again"; the cynical jokes of the nurses regarding "this time next year"; the undercurrent of hostility toward the nonsuffering fathers. I became unspeakably grateful that I had found out about the psychoprophylactic method and glad that I could now tell other people about it with conviction. It was interesting that despite the national, cultural and even linguistic gulf that divided the patients in this hospital from the patients I had been with in the English maternity hospital, their conversations about their labors and the whole subject of childbirth were almost identical.

Finally, I was very fortunate to be able to give birth under optimum conditions. The labor was short and developed normally, the staff at the hospital were cooperative and no one interfered with what I was doing. I had a doctor who was enthusiastic about the method and unfailingly generous with his time and concern. I also had the invaluable assistance and presence of my husband during the training period and throughout labor and delivery.

INFORMATION ABOUT
LOCAL COURSES

*Information about local courses may be
obtained from:*

ASPO

>National Headquarters and New York City Chapter:
>164 West 79th Street
>New York, New York

>Lafayette Chapter:
>1528 Alabama Street
>Lafayette, Indiana

>Long Island Chapter:
>1520 Blue Spruce Lane
>Wantagh, New York

>Los Angeles Chapter:
>13231 Calcutta Street
>Sylmar, California

Affiliates of ASPO

>Connecticut CALM
>38 Bayberry Lane
>Westport, Connecticut

CEA of Greater St. Louis
2 Chafford Woods
St. Louis, Missouri

Salt Lake City CEA
St. Mark's Hospital
Salt Lake City, Utah

Other groups (those marked with an asterisk may soon become ASPO affiliates)

CWPEA
201-34 Snowden
Detroit, Michigan

*Childbirth Preparation Service
2659 Fairway Drive
Jackson, Michigan

*Franklin County Childbirth Association
Village Green
Greenfield, Massachusetts

*Pioneer Valley CEA
Bay Road
Amherst, Massachusetts

HOPE
5327 Imogene St.
Houston, Texas

Lamaze Association for Childbirth Preparation
Ann Arbor, Michigan

Washington Area Lamaze Childbirth Group
2610 Henderson Avenue
Wheaton, Maryland

SUGGESTED READING LIST

Childbirth: A Manual for Pregnancy and Delivery, by John S. Miller (New York; Atheneum, 1963).

Childbirth Without Pain, by Pierre Vellay (New York; Dutton, 1959).

Expectant Motherhood, by Nicholson J. Eastman (4th ed., rev.; Boston; Little, Brown, 1963).

The First Nine Months of Life, by Geraldine Flanagan (New York; Simon and Schuster, 1962).

Pregnancy and Birth: A Book for Expectant Parents, by Alan F. Guttmacher (New York; New American Library, 1957).

Thank You, Dr. Lamaze, by Marjorie Karmel (Philadelphia; Lippincott, 1959).

BIBLIOGRAPHY

BABKIN, B. P., *Pavlov* (Chicago; the University of Chicago Press, 1949).

BAUDELOCQUE, J. L., *Midwifery* (Philadelphia; Bartram and Reynolds, 1807).

BING, E. D., KARMEL, M., and TANZ, A., *A Practical Training Course in the Psychoprophylactic Preparation for Labor* (New York; 1961).

CUNY, H., *Ivan Pavlov,* translated by Patrick Evans (London; Souvenir Press, 1964).

DICK-READ, G., *Childbirth Without Fear,* 2d ed. (New York; Dell Publishing Co., 1962).

EASTMAN, N. J., and HELLMAN, L. M., *Obstetrics* (New York; Appleton-Century-Crofts, Inc., 1961).

GRAHAM, H., *Eternal Eve* (Garden City; Doubleday and Co., 1951).

GUERNSEY, H., *Obstetrics* (Philadelphia; F. E. Boericke, 1867).

HERTZ, J. H., translator, *The Pentateuch and Haftorahs,* Volume I (New York; 1941).

JAKOBOVITS, I., *Jewish Medical Ethics* (New York; Bloch Publishing Co., 1959).

JOHNSON, C. O., *Government in the United States* (New York; Thomas Y. Crowell Co., 1948).

KARMEL, M., *Thank You, Dr. Lamaze,* 1st ed. (Philadelphia; Lippincott, 1959).

MEAD, M., *Male and Female* (New York; William Morrow and Co., 1949).

PAVLOV, I. P., *Lectures on Conditioned Reflexes,* translated by W. Horsley Gantt (New York; International Publishers, 1928).

POPE PIUS XII, "On Painless Childbirth," *The Catholic Mind,* Vol. LIV, No. 1121, pp. 280–91.

VELLAY, P., *Childbirth Without Pain* (New York; E. P. Dutton and Co., 1960).

VELVOVSKY, I., *Painless Childbirth Through Psychoprophylaxis* (Moscow; Foreign Languages Publishing House, 1960).

Index